KU-543-338

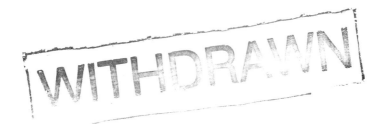

LIVERPOOL JMU LIBRARY

3 1111 01390 0947

Measuring Health and Wellbeing

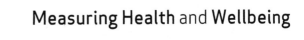

Titles in the Series

Leading for Health and Wellbeing ISBN 978 0 85725 290 6
Policy and Strategy for Improving Health and Wellbeing ISBN 978 0 85725 007 0
Assessing Evidence to Improve Population Health and Wellbeing ISBN 978 0 85725 389 7
Measuring Health and Wellbeing ISBN 978 0 85725 433 7

You can find more information on each of these titles and our other learning resources at
www.sagepub.co.uk

Measuring Health and Wellbeing

Editors:

John Harvey and Vicki Taylor

Series Editor:
Vicki Taylor

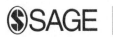

Los Angeles | London | New Delhi
Singapore | Washington DC

www.learningmatters.co.uk

Los Angeles | London | New Delhi
Singapore | Washington DC

www.learningmatters.co.uk

Learning Matters
An imprint of Sage Publications Ltd
1 Oliver's Yard
55 City Road
London EC1Y 1SP

SAGE Publications Inc.
2455 Teller Road
Thousand Oaks, California 91320

Sage Publications India Pvt Ltd
B 1/I 1 Mohan Cooperative Industrial Area
Mathura Road
New Delhi 110 044

SAGE Publications Asia-Pacific Pte Ltd
3 Church Street
#10-04 Samsung Hub
Singapore 049483

Editor: Alex Clabburn
Development editor: Ros Morley
Production controller: Chris Marke
Project management: Swales & Willis Ltd,
Exeter, Devon
Marketing manager: Tamara Navaratnam
Cover and text design: Wendy Scott
Typeset by: Swales & Willis Ltd, Exeter, Devon
Printed by: MPG Books Group, Bodmin, Cornwall

© John Harvey and Vicki Taylor, editors 2013

First published 2013

Apart from any fair dealing for the purposes of research or private study or criticism or review, as permitted under the Copyright, Designs and Patents Act, 1988, this publication may be reproduced, stored or transmitted in any form, or by any means, only with prior permission in writing of the publishers, or in the case of reprographic reproduction, in accordance with the terms of licences issued by the Copyright Licensing Agency. Enquiries concerning reproduction outside those terms should be sent to the publishers.

Library of Congress Central Number:
2012955071

British Library Cataloguing in Publication data:

A catalogue record for this book is available from the British Library

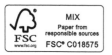

MIX
Paper from
responsible sources
FSC
www.fsc.org   FSC® C018575

ISBN 978 0 85725 832 8
ISBN 978 0 85725 433 7 (pbk)

Contents

Foreword from the Series Editor

The publication of the Public Health Skills and Career Framework in April 2008 provided, for the first time, an overall framework for career development in public health in the UK. Prior to this, the focus had been primarily on the public health specialist workforce. The development of the framework itself was a truly collaborative enterprise involving a large number of organisations and stakeholder groups and was designed to enable individuals at any stage of their career to identify a pathway for skills and career progression.

Within the framework, public health is divided into nine areas of work. There are four core areas that anyone working in public health must know about and have certain competences within. There are five non-core or 'defined' areas, representing the contexts within which individuals principally work and develop.

Core areas	Non-core (defined) areas
Surveillance and assessment of the population's health and wellbeing	Health improvement
	Health protection
Assessing the evidence of effectiveness of interventions, programmes and services	Public health intelligence
Policy and strategy development and implementation	Academic public health
Leadership and collaborative working	Health and social care quality

This new series, 'Transforming Public Health Practice', has been developed as a direct response to the development of the framework and has a book dedicated to each of the four core areas of public health. *Measuring Health and Wellbeing*; *Assessing Evidence to Improve Population Health and Wellbeing*; *Policy and Strategy for Improving Health and Wellbeing*; and *Leading for Health and Wellbeing* are all featured.

The framework defines nine levels of competence and knowledge. Level 1 will have little previous knowledge, skills or experience in public health, while those at level 9 will be setting strategic priorities and direction and providing leadership to improve population health and wellbeing. This series is aimed at those who want to develop their skills and knowledge in public health at levels 7–9 (which broadly equates to Master's level), although the series will be relevant to a wider group with the publication of the Public Health Practitioner standards and opening of the Public Health Practitioner Register (UKPHR). This will include those interested in acquiring or developing their public health competences and knowledge and, in particular, those who are seeking to demonstrate their public health skills and knowledge (and may be considering putting together a portfolio to demonstrate this, at specialist or practitioner level).

This series will also be useful for anyone whose work involves improving people's health and wellbeing, or has a direct impact on the health and wellbeing of communities and populations – this encompasses a wide range of work areas and of organisations and agencies.

Individual books in the series outline the key knowledge and skills in the core area and through case studies and scenarios show how these competences can be used in practice. Activities and self-assessment tools are provided throughout the book to help readers to hone their critical thinking and reflection skills.

Chapters in each of the books follow a standard format. At the beginning a box highlights links to relevant competences. This sets the scene and enables readers to see exactly what will be covered. This is extended by a chapter overview, which sets out the key topics and what readers should expect to have learnt by the end of the chapter.

There is usually at least one case study in each chapter, which considers public health skills and knowledge in practice. Activities such as practical tasks with learning points, critical thinking and reflective practice are included. Each activity is followed by a brief commentary on issues raised. At the end of each chapter a chapter summary provides a reminder of what has been covered.

All chapters are evidence-based in that they set out theory or evidence that underpins practice. In most chapters, one or more 'What's the evidence?' boxes provide further information. A list of additional readings is set out under the 'Going further' section, with all references collated at the end of the book.

In summary, this series will provide invaluable support to anyone studying or practising in the field of public health, in a range of different settings.

Vicki Taylor
Independent Public Health Consultant and Director
The Roundhouse Consultancy, MK Ltd
Associate Lecturer, The Open University
Previously Senior Lecturer, London South Bank University
Senior Lecturer, Kings College, London

Author Information

Claire Bradford graduated from Nottingham University Medical School in the 1980s and pursued a clinical career as a haematologist. She subsequently trained and worked in Public Health in the North East of England. Her appointments have included Director of Public Health in Newcastle upon Tyne and deputy director at the North East Public Health Observatory. Her professional interests include knowledge management, maternal and child health and reduction in health inequalities.

John Harvey is currently a director of a limited company providing public health consultancy. He trained as a public health consultant after working for nine years in the Yemen doing mainly maternal and child health programmes. He has experience as Director of Public Health in three different settings – Newcastle upon Tyne, Jersey and the London borough of Havering, where he was a visiting professor of public health at London South Bank University. He is an honorary Fellow of the Royal College of Paediatrics and Child Health. He was the co-chair (for the Faculty of Public Health) of the Child Public Health Interest Group for several years.

Mike Lavender currently works for NHS County Durham and Darlington. After medical qualification and junior doctor posts, he trained as a general practitioner. For the next 8 years he worked for different health programmes in Nepal, initially as a clinician but with increasing involvement in community health projects. On his return to the UK he trained in public health. He has been a consultant and doctor of public health in the North East since then, apart from another recent 2-year spell in Nepal.

Vicki Taylor has worked in public health since 1985 in a range of different roles at local, regional and national levels, and is now Director of the Roundhouse Consultancy MK Ltd, which offers consultancy in public health and leadership and management. She has a strong interest in public health development and, in particular, the development of public health leadership and management. She has substantive experience of public health and public health practitioner development in a number of geographical areas, spanning a period of more than 25 years. Vicki is Vice Chair of the UK Public Health Register (UKPHR) Registration Panel and is also an assessor for the UKPHR with experience of assessing public health portfolios at consultant (generalist specialist and defined specialist) and practitioner level. Currently she is providing learning sets and support for the West Midlands Public Health Practitioner's Assessment Scheme and the Surrey and Sussex Public Health Practitioner's Assessment Scheme and provided Commentary Writing Workshops support for the Public Health Practitioner Portfolio Development scheme in Wales.

Vicki provided learning sets to support the Kent and Medway Public Health Practitioner's Pilot Assessment Scheme and was the project manager for the NHS South Central public health practitioner development scheme from March 2007 until November 2009. In these roles Vicki has influenced and championed the development of public health practitioner schemes.

Rhonda Ware is a registered nurse who has worked at a senior level in the commercial, charity, local authority and health sectors, including private and the NHS. Rhonda was a senior manager in public health, having previous expertise in children's health and education, learning disabilities and care of the elderly. She is now Co-Director of Tiger Health Limited, which offers consultancy in healthcare and public health. Rhonda has a particular interest in leadership and change management, governance and quality improvement.

Acknowledgements

The editors would like to thank Rhonda Ware, Claire Bradford and Mike Lavender for their contributions to the text. Chapter 2 was written by John Harvey with contributions to the activities from Vicki Taylor. Chapter 3 was written by Mike Lavender with contributions from Vicki Taylor who wrote the sections on 'A five step approach to HNA and Rapid participatory appraisal' and activities 3.3 and 3.4.

The editors and publisher would like to thank the following for permission to reproduce copyright material:

Stockholm Institute for Future Studies for Figure 1.2; from Dahlgren and Whitehead (1991) *Policies and Strategies to Promote Social Equity in Health*.

Dr Rida Elkheir for *Health Needs Assessment: A Practical Approach* (2007).

The *British Medical Journal* for Wright, J, Williams, R and Wilkinson, JR (1998) Development and importance of health needs assessment. *BMJ*, 316:1310–1313.

The *British Medical Journal* for Murray, SA (1999) Experiences with 'rapid appraisal' in primary care: involving the public in assessing health needs, orientating staff, and educating medical students. *BMJ*, 318:440.

Every effort has been made to trace all copyright holders within the book, but if any have been inadvertently overlooked the publisher will be pleased to make the necessary arrangements at the first opportunity.

Introduction
Vicki Taylor

This book explores the knowledge and skills required to undertake meaningful measures of health and wellbeing.

One of the most important tasks we have as a society is to promote the health and wellbeing of our population, looking to improve their long-term quality of life. To do this we must understand two main issues: what determines health and wellbeing and how that influences the needs of any given population; and what impact interventions, whether a public health programme, a new social policy, a housing development or a health and social care service, have on individuals and the population – so-called outcomes. This understanding is informed by measuring health and wellbeing.

This is a vital aspect of public health practice. The practitioner must be able to plan and undertake straightforward need assessment for a local community or wider population. This requires a knowledge of how different measures are produced, the competence to give relevant interpretation of those measures and the skill to present the information in a compelling way.

Is this book for me?

This book is one of a series of four books aimed at addressing the core standards for public health practice as set out in the UK Public Health Skills and Career Framework (2008). It covers the first core area in the Public Health Skills and Career Framework: 'Surveillance and assessment of the population's health and wellbeing'.

Bringing together a basic understanding of need and measures used to express need and methods for doing health needs assessment (HNA) this book provides a practical resource that can be applied to public health and health promotion practice. It aims to make accessible from the vast health surveillance and population assessment literature some key concepts that may have relevance to measuring health and wellbeing. Through the use of case studies and activities, this book seeks to support the achievement of health improvement and health promotion goals. It is hoped that the approach taken gives the reader an opportunity to consider ways of contributing to the surveillance and assessment of the population's health and wellbeing.

The primary aim of the authors is to create a practical resource to support anyone preparing a portfolio for submission for registration as a defined specialist (at level 8), or registration as a public health practitioner (at level 5) and for those who are interested in the standards for measuring and surveying population health.

How the book works

This book is organised into six chapters. A consideration of the links between, and relative importance of, the various determinants of health and wellbeing is at the heart of Chapter 1. Chapter 2 introduces different types of measures and methods of measuring health and wellbeing and considers the difference between a measure and an indicator. Chapter 3 explores the notion of HNA as a means for identifying and prioritising the health needs of a community or population group. The chapter goes on to set out different approaches to carrying out an HNA, in particular the epidemiological approach and a five-step method. In Chapter 4 the emphasis shifts to health surveillance and what is required to establish an effective system for carrying out health surveillance. Health outcomes measurement and assessment are considered in Chapter 5.

The final chapter aims to provide the reader with a practical view of the use of measures of health and wellbeing to influence decision making, whether by commissioners or in a local strategic partnership. The chapter aims to provide models for practice and brings several strands together in a focus on tackling health inequalities.

How to use this book

You may be using this book to help prepare a portfolio for registration as a defined specialist (at level 8), for registration as a public health practitioner (at level 5) or as part of your studies. Once you are clear about the focus or standard you wish to consider, whether (for example) it is knowledge of methods for undertaking an HNA, look at the table below, which gives you a quick guide to the chapter titles and the standards (UK Public Health Skills and Career Framework (Department of Health 2008) and National Occupational Standards) and Public Health Practitioner Standards covered within the chapter. A chapter overview, at the beginning of each chapter, augments this information and sets you in the right direction.

Table 0.1 Chapters, UK Public Health Skills and Career Framework (PHSCF), National Occupational Standards (NOS) and Public Health Practitioner Standards (PHPS)

Chapter	PHSCF (knowledge and skills)		NOS	PHPS
1. Basic concepts	5g, 6d	5.5, 7.1	PHP10	6b
2. Measures of health and wellbeing	5c, 5d, 5f, 6c	5.2, 5.5	PHP10 PHP11	6a, 6b, 6c
3. Doing a health needs assessment	6c, 6d, 6e, 7a	5.1, 7.1, 7.6, 8.2	PHP08 PHP10 PHP11	6a, 6b, 6c
4. Health surveillance	5c, 5e, 6a	5.1, 6.3, 7.6.	PHP05	6b, 6c
5. Measuring health outcomes	5d, 6c, 7a, 7c	5.5, 7.2, 7.6	PHP05	6a, 6b, 6c
6. Intelligent application: defining the 'so-whats'	5a, 5d, 6c, 6d, 6e	5.2, 5.5, 5.6, 6.3, 7.1, 8.3	PHP04, PHP05, PHP06, PHP10, PHS02	6a, 6b, 6c

Notes:

Occupational standards are all related to core area 1, 'Surveillance and assessment of the population's health and wellbeing'.

PHP, Public Health Practice; PHS, Public Health Specialists – restructured 2007.

chapter 1

Basic Concepts

John Harvey

Meeting the Public Health Competences

This chapter will help you to evidence the following competences for public health (Public Health Skills and Career Framework):

- Level 5(g): Understanding of basic terms and concepts used in epidemiology and how rates are calculated;
- Level 5(5): Interpret data on health and wellbeing within own area of expertise or practice;
- Level 6(d): Understanding of links between, and relative importance of, the various determinants of health and wellbeing and needs;
- Level 7(1): Assess and describe the health and wellbeing and needs of specific populations and the inequities in health and wellbeing experienced by populations, communities and groups.

This chapter will also assist you in demonstrating the following National Occupational Standard for public health:

- Collect and link data and information about the health and wellbeing and related needs of a defined population (PHP10).

This chapter will also be useful in demonstrating Standard 6 of the Public Health Practitioner Standards.

Standard 6

Obtain, verify, analyse and interpret data and/or information to improve the health and wellbeing outcomes of a population/community/group – demonstrating:

b. knowledge of the main terms and concepts used in epidemiology and the routinely used methods for analysing quantitative and qualitative data.

Overview

This chapter will help you to understand links between, and relative importance of, the various determinants of health and wellbeing and need. It will also give you an understanding of basic terms and concepts used in epidemiology and how rates are calculated.

After reading this chapter you will be able to:

- define health and wellbeing, and needs assessment;
- understand that there are links between social determinants and health;
- describe what is involved in a joint strategic needs assessment (JSNA);
- define some key epidemiological and health economics concepts.

Introduction

One of the most important tasks we have as a society is to promote the health and wellbeing of our population, looking to improve their long-term quality of life. To do this we must have a good understanding of the needs of that population, whether children and young people, younger or older adults.

It is not just about 'data'. We also must involve people in a meaningful dialogue about their perceptions of need. It has been said that:

> experts and professionals can put their own interest before the wellbeing of their clients and research subjects. Often too they will be so ignorant of the reality of life for ordinary people that their proposals can be counter productive or just plain stupid.
>
> (Gough, 1992)

So we need to answer three basic questions. What is health and wellbeing? What determines health and wellbeing? What is need? We will answer the second question in discussing need and need assessment.

In addition, in this chapter we will review basic epidemiological and health economics principles and concepts so that you can assess the usefulness of all the available data.

What is health and wellbeing?

The World Health Organization (WHO) defined *health* as a state of complete physical, mental and social wellbeing and not merely the absence of disease or infirmity (WHO, 1948).

In 1986 this definition was revised for the *Ottawa Charter for Health Promotion*: *health* is seen as a resource for everyday life, not an object of living. It is a positive concept emphasising social and personal resources as well as physical capabilities – the extent to which an individual or group of individuals is able, on the one hand, to realise aspirations and satisfy needs, and on the other hand to change or cope with the environment (WHO, 1986).

Wellbeing is a term that is used increasingly in UK government policy. This may be to distinguish between the responsibilities of the health service and the wider joined-up approach to improving the status of the population. It is included in the original WHO definition to indicate much more than just a state of physical health. It also encompasses emotional stability, clear thinking, the ability to love, create, embrace change, exercise intuition and experience a continuing sense of spirituality. However wellbeing is defined in many ways in different contexts.

It has been suggested that the first and most important way to make sense of how *wellbeing* is used in contemporary policy is this: wellbeing is a *social construct*. There are no uncontested biological, spiritual, social, economic or any other kind of markers for wellbeing. The meaning of wellbeing is not fixed – it cannot be. It is a *primary cultural judgement*; just like *what makes a good life?* (Ereaut and Whiting, 2008).

What is need and needs assessment?

Need, in terms of healthcare, has been defined as the population's ability to benefit from health (and social) care interventions (Stevens and Raftery, 1994). Chapter 3 discusses needs assessment in more detail.

There are many models for the assessment of need in a population and health needs in particular. In this book, two approaches are recognised. The first approach starts with information gathered from different sources – these may be routine data from health surveillance, or local service use or applied rates from epidemiological studies in other populations – to identify aspects which are important or unusual in that population. In contrast, the second approach starts with a theoretical model which identifies the main factors that determine health and describes the local picture in the light of this. Both approaches will make use of the same sources of information (see Chapter 2 on measures of health) but the second aims to present the information in a way that illustrates the public health model. Taking this approach to assessment of need, there are two key models that have credibility and are mutually complementary: these are the life course and social determinants models.

The first is based on *life course theory*. Life course theories were developed to explain observations such as the way that the health of adults is influenced significantly by what they experienced during development both in the mother's womb and in their early years. The framework is described in a report entitled *Childhood Disadvantage and Adult Health: A Lifecourse Framework* (Graham and Power, 2004).

What's the evidence?

The life course framework provides an explanation for the persistence and worsening of inequalities by describing the ways in which health is transmitted from generation to generation. In the preface to the report (Graham and Power, 2004, pv), Kelly (then Director at the Health Development Agency) states that it is

> through economic, social and developmental processes, and the advantages and disadvantages are reinforced in adult life. A 'life-course approach' focuses on the different elements of the experience of health, from the moment of conception through childhood and adolescence to adulthood and old age.

There is very good evidence underpinning the importance and positive long-term outcomes of promoting early child development, through a range of services and interventions. The body of knowledge built up through longitudinal studies, based on life course theory, and informed by the understanding of developmental neurology (how the brain develops, for example) should be the basis of needs assessment.

The determinants of physical health and health behaviour are summed up in the preface to the report. Kelly goes on to say:

> disadvantaged childhood conditions have a direct impact on child health. So children from poorer circumstances tend to be affected in a number of ways: slower foetal growth, lower birth weight, shorter height and leg length, and more disease. Adolescence is critical in determining behaviour such as cigarette consumption, dietary behaviour, exercise and alcohol use, and while there is much evidence to show that children from all social groups tend to experiment with smoking and alcohol as well as drugs, the potentially damaging long-term use of drugs and alcohol, as well as consumption of fat, sugar and salt, are established in adolescence.
>
> (Graham and Power, 2004, pvi)

An example of the evidence to support this approach comes from the Northern Swedish Cohort Study (Gustafsson et al., 2011). This study is a prospective cohort study comprising all adolescents who entered or should have entered the ninth (last) grade of compulsory school in 1981 in a Swedish town. The influence of socioeconomic status (SES) on health over the life course is complex. Contrasting findings suggest that the enduring effect of childhood SES on adult body mass is largely independent of adult social class. This is known as the sensitive (or critical) period life course model, which suggests that exposure during particular periods of life (e.g. childhood/adolescence) results in long-term health effects, independently of later exposure. To understand the mediating factors and to determine how far this is true, a cohort study is the best method.

The Swedish study examined whether body mass index (BMI) at the age of 16, 21, 30 and 43 years, and 27-year BMI change, are explained by past and present socioeconomic disadvantage in women (and men), and if the SES–body mass association is explained by health behaviours. The results showed that, in women but not in men, associations between SES and body mass across the life course correspond to both the cumulative risk (persistently living in low SES) and sensitive period (in adolescence) models, and that health behaviours do not seem to mediate this association.

This important finding has implications: that to reduce social inequality in obesity in women, efforts should be directed at the early life course and not limited to targeting unhealthy behaviours.

However it is not only physical health but also social wellbeing which is explained by the life course framework. There are several ways in which this may be seen to work, and a model relating to social health is shown in Figure 1.1.

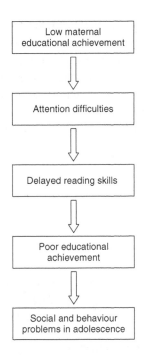

Figure 1.1 Model of social health

This model is drawn from cohort studies (Wickrama *et al.*, 2003) which show that, when a mother has a low educational achievement level, there is an increased likelihood that her child will show attention difficulties leading to delayed reading skills. This contributes to poor educational achievement by the child and this is associated with a higher risk of social and behavioural problems in adolescence.

Wickrama *et al.* (2003) illustrate this life course experience, showing how a combination of social disadvantage in the family of origin and adolescent maladjustment increases risk for physical health difficulties during adulthood. The results showed that early risk factors initiate a sequence of negative influences on young adult physical health through early entry into family responsibility, truncated educational attainment and poor occupational and economic status. These associations prevailed even after controlling for physical health status during adolescence.

The second model describes the influences on health and wellbeing – often called the social determinants of health – as the conditions in which people are born, grow, live, work and age. These conditions combine to influence wellbeing and are dependent on the quality of housing, education, employment and, for example, a nurturing environment in childhood. The negative influences associated with poverty are twofold:

1. People living in poverty are more likely to be exposed to conditions that are adverse to their health (crowded living conditions, unsafe neighbourhoods).

2. People living in poor circumstances are more likely to be negatively affected by these adverse conditions.

These influences have been described recently in the global examination of the social determinants of health (WHO, 2008a). Inequities in health are related to social and economic policies that lead generally to better health for those with higher incomes and better education. Once societies reach the level of affluence found in developed countries, further improvements in absolute standards make little difference to improving health. Differences in health at that stage begin to reflect differences in income distribution or income inequality, sometimes known as relative poverty, within each country. However the Commission on Social Determinants of Health emphasised a number of core influences at neighbourhood or community level:

- early child development and education;
- healthy places;
- fair employment;
- social protection;
- universal healthcare.

What's the evidence?

Social determinants of health: the solid facts

There are gross inequalities in health between countries. Life expectancy at birth, to take one measure, ranges from 34 years in Sierra Leone to 81.9 years in Japan. Within countries, too, there are large inequalities – a 20-year gap in life expectancy between the most and least advantaged populations in the USA, for example (Marmot, 2005). A boy born and living in Manchester will have 7 years' less life expectancy than a boy born and living in Surrey (APHO, 2010a).

Because the causes of the causes are not obvious, the WHO commissioned a summary of the evidence on the social determinants of health. This was published as *The Solid Facts* (Wilkinson and Marmot, 2003). It had ten messages on the social determinants of health based on:

1. the social gradient;
2. stress;
3. early life;
4. social exclusion;
5. work;
6. unemployment;
7. social support;
8. addiction;
9. food;
10. transport.

The Solid Facts reviewed evidence from Europe, aimed mainly at reducing inequalities in health within countries. The Commission on the Social Determinants of Health (WHO, 2008a) reviewed evidence on the social determinants of health that are relevant to global health and health inequalities.

One recognised illustrative picture of the interrelationships of the social determinants of health is shown in Figure 1.2 (see also Chapter 4 in the book *Leading for Health and Wellbeing* in this series). This picture (also known as Dahlgren and Whitehead's social model of health) makes clear the wide range of determinants that influence health. Age, gender and genetic constitution are at the centre. These inevitably influence people's health potential but are fixed. The next layer is related to individual lifestyle factors and ways of living that have the potential to promote or damage health. The third layer is social and community influences and networks. These can provide mutual support for members of the community but they can also provide no support or have a negative effect. The fourth layer focuses on general socioeconomic, cultural and environmental influences. These include structural factors such as housing, working conditions, agriculture and food production, access to services and provision of essential facilities.

Many of the *causes of the causes* of poor health and wellbeing, which probably account for 80 per cent of improvement in life expectancy, can be influenced locally, mainly through the local agencies acting in partnership.

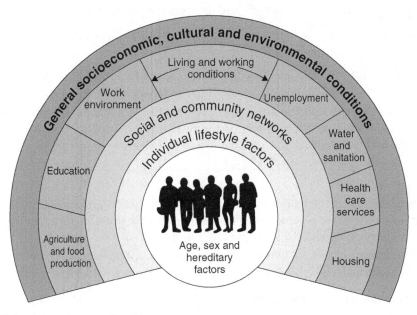

Figure 1.2 Wider determinants of health

Source: Dahlgren and Whitehead, 1991. Reproduced with permission from Institute for Futures Studies, Stockholm, Sweden.

Most determinants are included as domains in the Index of Multiple Deprivation (IMD) and nearly all indicators of health and wellbeing are predicted by this index (see Chapter 2). The IMD is a national measure of deprivation used in the UK.

ACTIVITY 1.1

Looking at the model of the determinants of health in Figure 1.2, what are the top five factors that have a negative impact on your community? What five factors have a positive effect on your community? Now look at the report published by the Marmot Review Team in 2010, *Fair Society, Healthy Lives* (access at: **www. marmotreview.org**) – does that change your selection?

Comment

In this exercise you are being asked to think about what you know about your community, which could be where you live or in public health terms the population whose health you work to improve. You might have identified employment as one of the key determinants that has a positive or negative effect. For example, if there has been a big change in the local economy such as the demise of an industry providing lots of jobs, then you would see redundancy and unemployment as a negative effect. On the other hand, if there was a new enterprise employing young people and school leavers, reducing the proportion of people aged 16–25 who are not in work or training, then this would be identified as a positive impact.

Taking another determinant, you might point to lifestyle factors such as binge drinking as a particular problem.

The Marmot Review will help identify factors which contribute positively to the life course and to reducing inequity. These may be the same – employment is a consistent theme, for example. However you may want to place emphasis on other themes. You would not select, say, some of the health-related indicators as factors but rather be clear about those causes of ill health which are important locally.

As needs assessment includes the ability to benefit from health (and social) care interventions, there has to be a process which identifies relative priorities for investment, as resources are not available to meet every need.

Priority frameworks set out the criteria to be used to rank different options for improving health and wellbeing. They focus on a number of concepts, such as:

- health outcome (how much benefit will this give to the individual?);
- health impact (how much benefit will this bring across the population?);
- clinical effectiveness (what is the probability of getting the desired effect?);
- cost-effectiveness (what does it cost to gain a quality-adjusted year of life?);
- evidence (how good is the evidence?);
- equity/non-discrimination (does it address inequity in provision or access?);
- access (does it improve access to the population as a whole?);
- autonomy/patient choice (does it allow or increase patient choice?).

Prioritisation and these frameworks are discussed in more detail in Chapter 6.

What is a joint strategic needs assessment?

Joint strategic needs assessments (JSNAs) were introduced by the government in 2006 in a document called *The Commissioning Framework for Health and Wellbeing* (DoH, 2007a, Appendix A, p64). The Local Government and Public Involvement in Health Act 2007 subsequently required local authorities and primary care trusts (PCTs), from 1 April 2008, to work together to produce a JSNA, focusing on the health and wellbeing of their local community. It is defined as:

> *'a process that identifies current and future health and wellbeing needs in light of existing services, and informs future service planning taking into account the evidence of effectiveness'. JSNA identifies 'the big picture' in terms of the health and wellbeing needs and inequalities of a local population.*
>
> (DoH, 2007b, p7)

When the JSNAs were first required, they were meant to feed into a number of important local strategies and plans. These included:

- the Sustainable Community Strategy (SCS), informing the priorities and targets set by the Local Area Agreement, which is the delivery agreement for the SCS;

- the Children and Young People's Plan of the local children's trust;

- the Commissioning Strategic Plan of the PCT.

The JSNA should identify priorities for commissioners, including general practitioners or clinical commissioners, to help to specify desired outcomes, and help providers shape services to address needs. Commissioning decisions informed by the JSNA should lead to improved health and wellbeing and reduced inequalities at best value for all (Figure 1.3). An important aspect of the assessment would be to predict levels of need 3–5 years ahead.

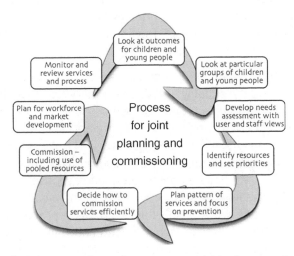

Figure 1.3 The place of a joint strategic needs assessment within the commissioning cycle

Source: Department for Children, Schools and Families and Department of Health, 2009. Reproduced under the terms of the Crown Copyright PSI Licence C2010000141.

A JSNA provides basic information about the needs of the population and should contain as wide a range of information as possible, whether addressing the needs of the whole population or the needs of a particular group, such as children and young people. What you should find is that the authors have used the most recent information available, and will have commonly used rates or trends (such as the annual rates shown over several years) to draw comparisons. These comparisons may be:

- within the area (comparing electoral wards, for example);
- with similar areas;
- with the national rate;
- with international rates.

What's the evidence?

The duty to produce a JSNA (HM Government, 2008)

Section 116 of the Sustainable Communities Act 2007 introduced the requirement for PCTs and responsible local authorities to produce a JSNA of the health and social care needs of their local community. It was envisaged that this assessment should set out the future health and social care needs of the local population. The assessment should cover those issues where the responsibilities of the PCTs and local authorities overlap, or where one organisation in carrying out its functions impacts to a significant extent on the other organisation's functions.

JSNAs consider the needs of the population living within the boundaries of the upper-tier local authority or unitary council. In two-tier local authority areas, upper-tier local authorities are required to consult with those district councils within their geographical area. In order to provide a firm link between the results of the JSNA and the SCS of each local authority, PCTs within a local authority's geographical boundary feed into a single assessment.

This guidance was superseded by new guidance from the Department of Health (2011a), giving Health and Wellbeing boards the primary responsibility for producing the JSNA. Recent draft guidance and current consultation propose, from April 2013, giving Health and Wellbeing boards the primary responsibility for producing the JSNA and joint health and wellbeing strategies (JHWSs), the strategies for meeting the needs identified in the JSNA. Local authorities, together with clinical commissioning groups, will have an equal and joint responsibility for producing the JSNA and JHWS. The local board is envisaged as the means for local government to work in partnership with commissioning groups to produce comprehensive JSNAs leading to the development of joint health and wellbeing strategies (Figure 1.4). These strategies therefore form the local framework for commissioning, including wider-ranging local interventions to address the determinants of health and wellbeing.

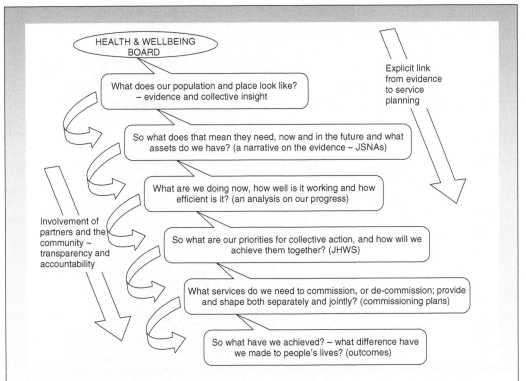

Figure 1.4 How joint strategic need assessments (JSNAs), joint health and wellbeing strategies (JHWSs) and commissioning plans fit together

Source: Department of Health (2012). Reproduced under the terms of the Crown Copyright PSI Licence C2010000141.

The draft guidance (Department of Health, 2012) emphasises the point that use of JSNAs is much more than simply a legal duty. Rather, it should be seen as an opportunity to develop the strategic framework to tackle need and inequalities in health and wellbeing at a local level. The new national emphasis is on improving life chances and outcomes for local communities, especially for people in the most vulnerable circumstances.

To do this it is expected that the JSNA will consider all current and future health and social care needs in relation to the area of the responsible authority. The guidance defines need as those factors (needs) which are capable of being met, or affected to a significant extent, by the local authority, clinical commissioning group or NHS Commissioning Board functions. This is in the context of preparing enhanced JSNAs, which must involve people living or working in the area.

Case Study: Key points from a joint strategic needs assessment

This box highlights some key points from the JSNA in a London borough about the local determinants of health.

Housing

- People aged 65 and over in the borough are more likely to be in accommodation with no central heating (22.3 per cent) than those in England (9.78 per cent).
- 53.6 per cent of council dwellings fell below the decent home standard, compared with 32.3 per cent for London and 26.2 per cent for England.
- Housing markers of poverty (homelessness, no central heating) are higher in the borough; this is especially noticeable among people aged 65 and over.
- 16 per cent of households are overcrowded. At 1 April 2009, the borough had a total of 6,154 overcrowded households wanting to be rehoused, of which 51 per cent were categorised as being severely overcrowded.[1]

Safety and crime

- Notifiable offence rates mirror geographic trends for deprivation, where the southern (132) and central (144) parts of the borough have higher rates per 1,000 population compared with the northern part (100). Youth gangs follow the same geographical pattern.
- Violent crime in the borough is above the England average. The level of the population exposed to violent crime is higher (3.7 per cent) than for England (1.4 per cent).
- Domestic violence rates in the borough are the 11th highest in the Metropolitan police service.
- One-third of notifiable offences in the borough were committed by young people under 19 years; reported crimes for children aged 10–17 are above the average for England.

Education

- Completed education attainment influences an adult's ability to provide for his/her family.

1 Occupancy rating of −2 or less (shortfall of bedrooms required for numbers in house).

Of the total population of the borough:

- 28.5 per cent have no educational or skills qualification;
- 41.5 per cent have level 1–3 qualifications;
- 24 per cent have a qualification of level 4/5;
- current levels of academic achievement are similar to those for England.

Key point

Higher educational attainment is linked to many beneficial behaviours and good health outcomes. Education offers opportunities for significant improvements in life expectancy and inequalities. While increases in education will take years to have an impact, the impact will affect people's lives for years.

ACTIVITY 1.2

Health profiles for local authorities are produced annually by the Association of Public Health Observatories (funded by the Department of Health). Find the profile for your population (accessed at **www.apho.org.uk**).

What does it tell you about the determinants of health?

Does the profile identify any particular need that you would want to highlight (remember – is there the ability to benefit?)

Prepare a summary of 100 words to present to your local Health and Wellbeing board.

Comment

The guidance defines need as those factors (needs) which are capable of being met, or affected to a significant extent, by commissioners. In this case you will want to present something giving one or two priorities which can be positively affected by the actions of the Health and Wellbeing board, collectively or through individual partners.

If one of the key issues is the levels of domestic violence (see case study above), you would explain briefly why it is a local priority, what might be contributing to the problem and what interventions could be put in place.

The core dataset

The case study shows a variety of information about housing, safety and education. Previous guidance from the Department of Health included the publication of a JSNA core dataset in 2008 to aid local authorities and PCTs in the process. This

LIVERPOOL JOHN MOORES UNIVERSITY
LEARNING SERVICES

national dataset proposes use of approximately 250 key indicators, including 68 top-level measures, which can be used to compare one area with others. Indicators or measures like these are discussed in the next chapter.

The core dataset provides an indicative list of indicators to assist partnerships in preparing their JSNA in several domains. Further information on each indicator is provided either within the guidance or in the official *Handbook of Definitions* for the national indicator set. This was updated in April 2009 (see **www.yhpho.org.uk**) and the core dataset now contains additional national indicators and vital signs (the NHS equivalent).

The indicators are divided into *domains* and *sub-domains*. These are not official categories. The domains include demography, social and environmental context and burden of ill health. The 'demography' domain underpins the JSNA, both by setting local context and as an essential component in producing projections and break-downs of need. The remaining domains, sub-domains (and sub-sub-domains) con-tain indicators which either measure need or are a proxy for it. Some of them relate to a particular age group. Many are related to factors such as housing and employ-ment; on the other hand, some are disease-specific.

There are many sources of data. Here are the websites for various sources which are referred to in Chapter 2, where we describe specific measures.

- Office for National Statistics (**www.statistics.gov.uk**);
- Hospital Episode Statistics (**http://www.hesonline.nhs.uk**);
- Association of Public Health Observatories (**www.apho.org.uk**);
- Communicable diseases (**www.hpa.org.uk**);
- Quality Management and Analysis System (**www.pcc.nhs.uk/qmas**);
- National Cancer Intelligence Network (**www.ncin.org.uk**);
- Clinical and Health Outcomes Knowledge Base (**http://nchod.uhce.ox.ac.uk/**);
- Prescribing data (**www.ic.nhs.uk/statistics-and-data-collections/primary-care/prescriptions**);
- Mental Health Profiles (**www.erpho.org.uk/pub/mhp09.aspx**);
- Compendium of Clinical and Health Indicators (**http://indicators.ic.nhs.uk**).

Addressing inequalities

The JSNA should focus upon the inequalities in the local area, and identify those groups which are getting a 'raw deal'. Demographic indicators which could provide a useful breakdown for the study of inequality in other indicators are marked in the dataset. For instance, a particular need may be higher or lower in certain age groups or ethnic groups, among disabled people or in deprived areas.

Methods of analysing and expressing inequalities in health and wellbeing are described in part 5 of JSNA – the APHO Resource Pack, Measuring Health Inequalities (APHO, 2008). The challenge of reducing inequalities is addressed in Chapter 6.

The next section in this chapter will consider some of the key epidemiological concepts used in measuring health and wellbeing.

Key epidemiological concepts

This is not an epidemiological textbook, but epidemiology underpins our knowledge of the models of the determinants of health and wellbeing, and will help answer some important questions. Understanding some key concepts will help make sense of the abundance of data which is available.

Epidemiology is the study of the natural history of disease in a population. It seeks to understand the causes, distribution and control of disease in populations.

A *causative agent* may cause disease by its presence (e.g. common cold virus) or absence (e.g. lack of vitamin D). Broadly, epidemiologists look at the relationship between aspects of the total environment in which individuals live and outcomes over time. Those environmental factors include the physical environment, the socio-economic context and/or the biological influences. It is possible to measure the impact of these factors on susceptible or 'at-risk' individuals and groups and predict a level of risk in respect of the probability of developing a specific condition, or probability of death.

Distribution requires some measure of frequency – how often and how many cases in the population. An important principle is that epidemiology is looking at disease outcomes in a specified population – the population at risk.

The classical types of study are descriptive – cross-sectional, cohort or case-control studies; or interventional – a clinical or community trial.

A *cross-sectional* study examines the relationship between diseases or other aspects of health and variables such as exposure to risk factors in a defined population at one particular time.

A *cohort* study examines multiple health effects (positive or negative) of an exposure. An exposure may be a social or environmental factor, or a lifestyle factor. Subjects are followed over time and analysis is defined according to their exposure levels and future occurrence of disease or other health effects. A cohort study will define disease incidence because you can count how many specific events (such as people being diagnosed with diabetes) occur in the cohort each year.

A *case-control* study examines multiple exposures in relation to a disease or particular condition. Those subjects with the condition are defined as cases and then matched with controls who do not have the condition. Matching is usually done on age and gender and exposure histories of cases and controls are then obtained and compared.

An *interventional* or *experimental* study, also known as a trial, investigates the role of some agent in the prevention or treatment of a disease. In this type of study, individuals are assigned to two or more groups that either receive or do not receive the intervention, i.e. an intervention group and a comparison group.

An *ecological* study is an epidemiological study in which the unit of analysis is a population rather than an individual. For instance, an ecological study may look at the association between smoking and lung cancer deaths in different countries.

Bias is a systematic tendency to over- or under-estimate the number of cases or events. This may occur for different reasons. The individuals or populations studied (or responding) may not be representative of the population, the information source may be incomplete (e.g. because some cases have not been notified) and the measurement used may be inconsistent. Much of our information comes from counting events, which are measured for strategic (often mandatory) purposes or operational reasons and we need to be aware of the limitations.

Other key terms used in epidemiology are incidence and prevalence. *Incidence* is the rate at which new cases (or events) occur in a population in a specified period. For example, incidence of bowel cancer is the number of new cases of bowel cancer which occur in a year for every 100,000 of the population.

Prevalence is the proportion of the population who are cases at a point in time. This could be the percentage of people who smoke, or the percentage of people who have ever been diagnosed with diabetes.

In order to ensure consistency, and enable comparison, the *case* must be clearly defined. For example, if we want to know the prevalence of asthma in children then counting those who have been given a diagnostic label of asthma may miss children who have symptoms which are characteristic (such as waking at night with wheezing) but who are not labelled as asthmatic.

The number of cases determines the nominator in calculating *rates*, i.e. the number to be divided by the number in the population at risk, or the denominator. The denominator is the lower part of a fraction used to calculate a rate or ratio; in a rate, the denominator is usually the population, or population experience, as in person-years, at risk. Care needs to be taken to ensure the nominator is related to the appropriate 'at-risk' population.

Incidence and prevalence are common types of rates, as are mortality rates, which are usually expressed as rates for a specific disease or group of conditions. A simple calculation will produce what is called a *crude rate*. For example, if there are 2,000 deaths from all causes in a population of 200,000, the crude mortality rate is 10 per 1,000. Rates may be refined to make them more relevant or to be able to use them to make comparisons.

An overall rate for the population may disguise the fact that the incidence varies with age. For many conditions (e.g. cataracts) the incidence rises with age, so age-specific rates are helpful in planning and assessing change over time as the age structure of the population changes. These rates may also be better examined by gender.

To adjust rates to allow comparison between rates for different populations, the technique known as *standardisation* is used. The aim is to reduce the confounding factors such as age, gender and SES. Age is the common basis of standardisation.

There are two main standardisation methods, characterised by whether the standard used is a population distribution (direct method) or a set of specific rates (indirect method). The direct method is used to calculate a *standardised rate*, which can be compared properly with the standardised *rate* for another population. A common use in England is the standardised hospital admission rate for different conditions.

The indirect method is used to calculate a standardised *ratio*, so the frequency of events in the population is effectively compared to the standard population. The *standardised mortality ratio* (SMR) is calculated by dividing the total of observed deaths by the total of expected deaths. The number of expected deaths is calculated by applying age-specific rates for the standard population to the target population age groups. If it is greater than 1 (or 100 if expressed as a percentage), it indicates that the risk of dying in the observed population is higher than what would be expected if it had the same experience or risk as the standard population. On the other hand, a SMR lower than 1 (or 100) indicates that the risk of dying is lower in the observed population than expected if its distribution were the same as the reference population.

In the following case studies we are going to calculate age-standardised rates and SMRs.

Case Study: Calculating standardised mortality ratios

Directly age-standardised rate for deaths from all circulatory diseases (ICD10 I00–I99, ICD9 390–459)[2] for males aged under 75 years

Stage 1: Calculate the age-specific rates in area A

You need to know two things – the number of events (deaths) by age group in area A for a given year (or over a number of years, e.g. a 3-year average). The narrower the age group the better. Five-year age bands are suggested here. The second set of data you need are the numbers of the population in each age group in area A. Now divide the number of deaths (row a) by the population (row b), and multiply by 100,000 to calculate the age-specific rate.

	Sex	0–1	1–4	5–9	...	65–69	70–74
a. Observed events (deaths)	M	0	0	0	...	50	70
b. Population	M	2,200	9,300	11,900	...	5,800	4,700
c. Age-specific rates per 100,000 ((a/b) × 100,000)	M	0.0	0.0	0.0	...	862	1489

2 The *International Classification of Disease* (ICD) has had many revisions. The commonly used version in the UK is ICD10, but ICD9 is still in use in some information systems.

Stage 2: Calculate the expected number of events (deaths) in the standard population, given the age-specific rate in area A

The standard European population is a fixed standard with numbers of population by age group and by gender. These numbers go in row d. The age-specific rates for area A are now put in row e. These rates are expressed as numbers per 100,000, but to be applied will have to be divided by 100,000. (The rates could have been left as decimal rates, e.g. 0.01489 for the 70–74 age group.) This calculation gives you the number of expected deaths per age group (row f).

Age group	0	1–4	5–9	...	65–69	70–74
d. Standard population (European standard population) by age group	1,600	6,400	7,000	...	4,000	3,000
e. Age-specific rates of area A	0.0	0.0	0.0	...	862	1,489
f. Expected number of events (deaths) in the standard population ((e) × (d))/ 100,000)	0.00	0.00	0.00	...	34	45

Stage 3: Calculate the age-standardised annual rate

Add up the total expected events across all appropriate age groups (row f) to give a total number of expected events for the year selected (column aa). Add up the standard population across all the selected age groups (row d) and put the total in column bb. Divide the total expected events (aa) by the total standard population (bb) and multiply by 100,000 to give the age-standardised rate. Note that the total used here (column aa) is illustrative rather than actual.

aa. Total expected deaths 0–74 years	bb. Total standard population 0–74 years	Standardised rate 0–74 years
140	96,000	145.83

i.e. in area A the directly standardised rate for deaths from circulatory disease in males in that year was 146 per 100,000.

Case Study: Calculating standardised mortality ratios

Indirectly standardised rates compare the actual number of events in an area (e.g. South Gloucestershire) with the expected number of events based on mortality rates of a reference population (e.g. England and Wales).

This method is often used to look at differences in mortality rates, and is often referred to as the standardised mortality ratio (SMR). The SMR is a ratio of observed to expected number of deaths. It can also be used to look at other events, such as hospital activity, e.g. standardised admission rates. The observed figures come from the local area, and the expected figures from applying the death rate in the reference population to the local population.

Example

In this example we are comparing mortality in people aged 64 and younger in area A to mortality in England and Wales for the same age range. The actual number of deaths in area A was 560. The following steps are used to calculate the SMR.

Step 1

Find the age-specific death rates in the reference population, England and Wales, and put in column a. In this example the age bands are wider than in the case study using the direct standardisation method.

Step 2

Find the populations in area A for the same age bands, and put in column b.

Step 3

Calculate the expected deaths in each of the age groups by multiplying the population in area A by death rate in the reference population (England and Wales) and dividing by 100,000, i.e. expected deaths per 100,000 = (b × c)/100,000.

The table below shows the calculation of steps 1–3.

Step 1	Step 2	Step 3	
a	b	c	d
Age groups	Deaths per 100,000 in England and Wales	Population in area A	Expected deaths per 100,000
15–24	31	60,000	18.6
25–34	45	64,000	28.8
35–44	84	63,000	52.9
45–54	120	69,000	82.8
55–64	554	58,000	321.3

Step 4

Add up the number of deaths in each age group (column d) to get the total number of expected deaths. This total is 504.

Step 5

The SMR can now be calculated. It is the observed number of deaths/ expected number of deaths expressed as a percentage.

In this example, the SMR is (560/504) × 100 = 111.

When looking for comparisons to make a judgement about the relative importance of a rate, standardised ratios provide the comparison by reference to the standard population. Often it is the national rate which is used as the standard. Similarly, rates may be compared to a regional average, or an average for populations, which are treated as a cluster because they have similar characteristics (such as inner city or rural). The difficulty here is that the usual or average is not necessarily good and having a better (or worse) rate than average may divert attention from an unacceptably low or high value. Similarly, use of distributions of values and asking which percentile (often quintiles, i.e. every 20 per cent of the values) a given population comes into, may lead to false assumptions. Where possible it is good to have a true benchmark, set by either evidence or international agreement on excellence.

ACTIVITY 1.3

This activity gives you some real data to use to work through the methodology for standardisation. Go to the website for the Office for National Statistics (**www.ons. gov.uk**) and search for cancer incidence.

Choose the cancer incidence – results (by year) for Scotland. This will take you to the Information Services Department, NHS Scotland webpage. Download the data tables (in Excel) and you will have a menu of specific cancers or all cancers. Choose one table and you will find age-specific rates both for Scotland as a whole and for regions. Choose a region, and apply the rates to a standard European population, and compare your answer with the published rate. You can also check the standardised incidence ratio (same method as SMR) for the region compared against Scotland as the standard population.

Comment

There are many sources of data to help you do similar exercises until you are familiar with the method. You may find it helpful to ask a local public health analyst to check your working.

Key health economic concepts

Scarcity

This is where the total resources are not enough to provide for all the interventions which are available to meet the needs of the population, and there are no means of securing additional resources. Scarcity is a fundamental concept, and the need for health economic analysis stems from an understanding of the implications of the notion of scarcity.

Health status

This is the degree to which a person is able to function on a day-by-day basis physically, emotionally and socially. This concept is discussed in more detail in the chapter on outcomes (Chapter 5).

In order to compare the relative value of an intervention aimed at improving health status, some measure is needed which is independent of the specific medical condition and its effects, or the type of intervention. The common approach to this is to use a measure which combines life years gained as a result of health interventions/ healthcare programmes with a judgement about the quality of these life years. The *quality-adjusted life year* (QALY) is the commonly used measure.

Quality-adjusted life year

The QALY is a measure of disease burden, which takes account of both how much life is added (the quantity) and how the individual feels about his or her quality of life.

The QALY is based on the number of years of life that would be added by the intervention. A 'utility' value is assigned which ranges from 0.0 to 1.0. Each year in perfect health is assigned the value of 1.0. If the extra years would not be lived in full health, for example if the patient suffered chronic pain, or had severe visual impairment or had to use a wheelchair, then the extra life years are given a value between 0 and 1 to account for this.

Cost–benefit analysis (CBA)

CBA is an economic evaluation in which all the costs of providing an intervention and the consequences of a programme or intervention are expressed in the same units, usually money. CBA is used to compare costs and benefits across programmes serving different patient groups. Even if some items of resource or benefit cannot be measured in the common unit of account, i.e., money, they should not be excluded from the analysis. Costs would include use of resources beyond the costs falling on the health service alone, e.g. costs falling on other services such as social care or voluntary sector, costs to society such as loss of productivity and costs borne by patients and their carers.

Cost-effectiveness analysis (CEA)

CEA is an economic evaluation in which the costs of alternative interventions are expressed as cost per unit of health outcome, usually measured in QALYs. The incremental cost-effectiveness ratio (ICER) is now used as the first-line method of comparing cost-effectiveness. The results of the cost-effectiveness analysis are expressed by means of the ICER, which is defined as the ratio of the change in costs of a therapeutic intervention (compared to the alternative, such as doing nothing or using the best available alternative treatment) to the change in effects of the intervention. As a formula, for interventions A and B:

$$\text{ICER} = \text{costs (A)} - \text{costs (B)}/\text{QALYs (A)} - \text{QALYs (B)}$$
(Walker *et al.*, 2007)

Opportunity cost

Opportunity cost is the loss of potential gain, such as years of life or quality of life, for one group of the population which is foregone when a commissioner decides to invest in a programme or intervention for another population group. If, for example, a local authority can only afford to fund one of the following – an early years centre, or a centre of excellence for people with dementia – then the opportunity cost of choosing one can be seen to be the loss of the benefit that would have been delivered by the other.

Programme budgeting and marginal analysis (PBMA)

PBMA is a process that helps decision-makers maximise the impact of healthcare resources on the health needs of a local population. Programme budgeting is an appraisal of past resource allocation in specified programmes, with a view to tracking future resource allocation in those same programmes. The programmes are often categorised by clinical specialities, e.g. diseases of the circulation.

Marginal analysis is the appraisal of the added benefits and added costs of a proposed investment (or the lost benefits and lower costs of a proposed disinvestment) within the programme (Brambleby and Fordham, 2003).

Technical efficiency

Technical efficiency exists when a given level of output can be achieved with a minimal level of input. It is assessed by seeing whether the given output can be achieved by using less of one input while holding all other inputs constant. For example, is it more cost-effective for a consultant dermatologist, say, to go to primary care centres to do a clinic than have patients go to a hospital outpatients department?

Allocative efficiency

Allocative efficiency exists when no change in spending priorities could improve the wellbeing of one population group without reducing the wellbeing of another group.

Chapter summary

This chapter has introduced a number of definitions of health and wellbeing, and the concept of needs assessment. The links between determinants of health and wellbeing and need were considered. In reviewing what is meant by health and wellbeing and need, and need assessment, two frameworks were offered – a life course framework and the social determinants of health model. JSNA was introduced and the significance of the development of a JSNA in improving the health and wellbeing of a population was explored. The importance of a core dataset was emphasised, together with consideration of other sources of data that can be used to assist the preparation of JSNAs. Undertaking a needs assessment is discussed in more detail in Chapter 3.

A number of key epidemiological terms and concepts were introduced, including the calculation of age-standardised mortality ratios and SMRs, as this understanding is fundamental to interpreting the wealth of data available. The chapter concluded with some consideration of the most important health economic concepts.

GOING FURTHER

Coggon, D, Rose, G and Barker, DJP (1997) *Epidemiology for the Uninitiated*, 4th edn. London: BMJ Publishing Group.
This is a very readable guide to the theory, techniques and language of epidemiology.

Glasby, J and Ellins, J (2008) *Implementing Joint Strategic Needs Assessment: Pitfalls, Possibilities and Progress*. Health Services Management Centre, University of Birmingham. Available online at: **www.dh.gov.uk/en/Publicationsandstatistics/ Publications/PublicationsPolicyAndGuidance/DH_086130** (accessed 4 August 2012).
This report of a survey of PCTs and local authorities sets out the findings in regard to (then) current approaches, existing data and public and patient involvement. It examines the potential implications of JSNA and offers suggestions for practical support and how JSNAs could be the stimulus for longer-term change.

Napper, M and Newland, J (2002) *Health Economics Information Resources: A Self Study Course*. Available online at: **www.nlm.nih.gov/nichsr/edu/ healthecon/index.html**.
This self-study course comprising four modules describes the scope of health economics and information resources. Drawing on the US healthcare system it focuses on sources and characteristics of healthcare financing information in order to provide an overview and discussion of important sources of health economics information and enable the development of a good understanding of health economic principles.

Orme, J, Powell, J, Taylor, P, Harrison, T and Grey, M (eds) (2003) *Public Health for the 21st Century: New Perspectives on Policy, Participation and Practice*. Maidenhead: McGraw-Hill/Open University Press.
The chapter on epidemiology in the twenty-first century (Chapter 15), although a little demanding, highlights and points to some important ways in which the development of public health practice and epidemiology are interrelated. The chapter on health economics (Chapter 16) provides a more detailed discussion of the concepts outlined in this chapter.

chapter 2

Measures of Health and Wellbeing

John Harvey

Meeting the Public Health Competences

This chapter will help you to evidence the following competences for public health (Public Health Skills and Career Framework):

- Level 5(c): Knowledge of basic quantitative and qualitative methods of surveillance and assessment of the population's health and wellbeing;
- Level 5(d): Understanding of the relevance and use of measures of socioeconomic deprivation in population health and wellbeing analysis;
- Level 5(f): Knowledge of the strengths and weaknesses of various types of data relating to health and wellbeing and needs;
- Level 5(2): Analyse routine data on health and wellbeing and needs using basic analytical techniques;
- Level 5(5): Interpret data on health and wellbeing within own area of expertise or practice;
- Level 6(c): Understanding of strengths, uses, interpretation and limitations of various types of data relating to health and wellbeing, needs and outcomes.

This chapter will also assist you in demonstrating the following National Occupational Standards for public health:

- Collect and link data and information about the health and wellbeing and related needs of a defined population (PHP10);
- Analyse and interpret data and information about the health and wellbeing and related needs of a defined population (PHP11).

This chapter will also be useful in demonstrating Standard 6 of the Public Health Practitioner Standards.

Standard 6

Obtain, verify, analyse and interpret data and/or information to improve the health and wellbeing outcomes of a population/community/group – demonstrating:

a. knowledge of the importance of accurate and reliable data/information and the anomalies that might occur;
b. knowledge of the main terms and concepts used in epidemiology and the routinely used methods for analysing quantitative and qualitative data;
c. ability to make valid interpretations of the data and/or information and communicate these clearly to a variety of audiences.

Overview

This chapter looks at definitions and types of measures and methods of measuring health and wellbeing and should help you to understand the difference between a measure and an indicator. It addresses some of the issues you need to be familiar with to make good use of the various measures or indicators. We will discuss issues relating to different categories of measures which determine what we are measuring and consider what measures make good indicators. The various methods of measuring are described and key features that determine the quality of the data are outlined. A number of useful sources of information which were also listed in Chapter 1 are referred to throughout the chapter.

Exercises in this chapter will focus on:

• understanding what measures are frequently used in population health surveillance and what constitutes a 'good' indicator;
• understanding and choosing appropriate measures;
• understanding the issues involved in the quality of data.

This chapter uses theory, tools and case studies to appreciate some of the key indicators and measures that are used in the surveillance and assessment of the population's health and wellbeing.

After reading this chapter you will be able to:

• distinguish between an indicator and a measure;
• explain the use of indicators to investigate differences between populations;
• appreciate what constitutes a 'good' measure and have an understanding of different ways of measuring;
• know about routine sources of information.

Introduction

Surveillance and assessment of the population's health and wellbeing is one of the four core areas of public health work. This involves use of routine or available data to improve health. *Surveillance* is often used synonymously with *monitoring*. Health surveillance has a specific meaning and this is defined and discussed in Chapter 4. These data are usually presented in the form of measures or indicators. In order to make comparisons there needs to be agreement on how to collect the data and in determining what indicators are used. Where this is not done then it can be difficult to make comparisons across different datasets. Consider the findings of a study published in 2010 comparing the rates of self-reported health in different countries in Europe. The authors suggest indicators of poor health are generally higher than average in the metropolitan areas in the north and west of the UK and the central belt and south-east of Germany, and lower in the areas of Sweden generally and north-west Belgium. Variations between the socioeconomic composition of the local area populations do not explain these health differences. Another possible explanation is that the way the indicators were measured (by health surveys) in each country varies so that the comparisons are invalid to some extent (Gray *et al.*, 2012).

The steps needed to assure the quality of common datasets so that they may be used reliably for comparisons with and between areas or nations are discussed in Chapter 4. The two key elements are definition of the 'event' which is being counted, and robust data management.

Measures and indicators: is there a difference?

A measure will determine the dimensions, for example quantity or frequency, of a subject by use of a standard unit and may be used to draw comparison with a standard value. Weight and height are typical measures (how much is there?), as is incidence (how often does something happen?).

A health indicator is a type of measure. It expresses a characteristic of an individual, population or environment which is subject to measurement (directly or indirectly). It can be used to describe one or more aspects of the health of an individual or population, whether quality or quantity, and can be expressed in relation to a time period. If we combine weight and height using a formula (weight in kilograms/height in metres squared) we have a commonly used indicator, the body mass index, that is used to define obesity. Health indicators may include measures relating to the determinants of health and wellbeing. This could be the percentage of the population living in relative poverty or a measure of behaviours such as the percentage of people aged 16–25 who report drinking alcohol at a given level of units per week.

Health indicators can be used to define health problems at a particular point in

Table 2.1 Comparing performance indicators and measures

Indicators		Measures	
Indicators only indicate	Never completely capture the richness and complexity of a system; designed to give 'slices' of reality	Measures measure specific characteristics	Should be relevant and accurate in respect of the selected characteristic but are not necessarily indicative of the whole
Indicators encourage explicitness	Force us to be clear and explicit about what we are trying to do	Measures are specific and inherently explicit	Should be valid and timely, with common interpretation
Indicators usually rely on numbers and numerical techniques	In order to be able to use indicators properly or challenge them, we need a basic understanding of elementary statistics	Measures also rely on numbers and numerical techniques	Basic understanding of epidemiology and statistics is needed
Indicators should not just be associated with fault-finding	They can help us understand performance, be it good or bad	Measures can describe differences	Variation can be related to a standard Variation can be measured without indicating good or bad

Source: Adapted from APHO, 2008.

time; to indicate change over time in the level of the health of a population or individual; and to define differences in the health of populations. In summary, indicators are succinct measures that aim to describe as much as possible about a system (such as a health and social care service) or population in as few points as possible (AHPO, 2008). Indicators help us understand the issues, and to compare and measure change. Table 2.1 provides a comparison of performance indicators and measures.

ACTIVITY 2.1

Look at the following examples of measures that are frequently used in population health surveillance and their definitions and consider in turn whether each of these would make a 'good' indicator.

Why do you think this?

What is your justification for your decision?

Table 2.2 Examples of measures

Measure	Definition
Infant mortality	Number of deaths under 1 year old per 1,000 live births
Life expectancy	Years a male or female child born today would expect to live
Smoking	Prevalence as percentage of adult population (18+ years)
Childhood obesity	Prevalence as percentage of children at reception and year 6
Alcohol admissions	Number of alcohol-related admissions to hospital per 100,000 population
Accident mortality	Deaths from accidents per 100,000 population
Hip fractures in elderly	Number of hip fractures in people aged 65 and over per 100,000 population
Suicide rate	Numbers of suicides and undetermined deaths per 100,000
Dementia	Number of people on dementia register as percentage of general practitioner-registered population
GCSE	The percentage of students achieving 5 A*–C results, including English and maths
NEET	The percentage of young people aged 16–18 not in education, employment or training

Comment

Infant mortality, life expectancy, childhood obesity, hip fractures, suicide rates, GCSE rates (as the percentage of students achieving 5 A*–C results, including English and maths) and NEETs (the percentage of young people aged 16–18 not in education, employment or training) are generally considered to be good indicators. Infant mortality is historically used as a comparator at international level and life expectancy is now commonly used to highlight differences between populations. Childhood obesity is measured through the National Child Measurement Programme.

Smoking prevalence rates for local populations are 'synthetic estimates' from national surveys and the number of alcohol-related admissions to hospital per 100,000 population or 'alcohol admissions' acts as a proxy for the amount of 'problem' drinking in the population and as such are not considered to be 'good indicators'; however, in the absence of other measures they are used. Deaths from accidents per 100,000 of the population (or accident mortality rate) are limited if the specific types of accident (e.g. fire or drowning) are not separated. The number of people on the dementia register as a percentage of the general practitioner (GP)-registered population is typical of another sort of data problem, when the count depends on the proactive behaviour of the clinician in recognising and recording the diagnosis. Interestingly, the number of hip fractures in people aged 65 and over per 100,000 population assumes all fractures are admitted and is considered a good proxy for incidence. Understanding what is behind each of these measures is important in considering whether or not they are potentially 'good' indicators. A 'good' indicator is something which can accurately and reliably describe one or more aspects of the health of an individual or population.

What are we measuring?

Measures of health and wellbeing can be divided into four main categories: demographic measures, activity-based measures, output measures and outcome measures, including quality of life.

Demography is the study of human populations. This includes births, deaths, migration size, growth, density, distribution, age, gender and ethnicity. Social demographic measures expand on these and include income, disabilities, mobility (in terms of travel time to work or number of vehicles available), educational attainment, home ownership, employment status and marriage status.

Activity-based measures count people attending, or clients of, a facility or service, or undergoing a procedure or intervention. They tend to measure how busy or popular a facility is rather than absolute need. However, if an event requires an admission to hospital (such as an acute stroke), then it is probable the admission rate will approximate to the incidence of non-fatal stroke.

Outputs are the product of a process. An immunisation programme is a process which delivers a given vaccine to a proportion of the population. If 1,000 persons are eligible for the vaccine, the target population, and 860 are immunised, the output is 86 per cent. The actual outcome is twofold: the numbers who have had an adequate immune response and are resistant to the infection; and the numbers who did not have an adequate response plus the number who were not immunised – the susceptible.

An *outcome* is a measure of achievement. In health terms it is related to the change in health status of the individual or the relevant population group. In the example of the immunisation programme above, it is those resistant or immune and those who are still susceptible. Death is an outcome, as is full recovery on the other hand. Change in quality of life may be the most important outcome for many enduring conditions. Outcomes are discussed in Chapter 5.

Case Study: What measures are collected routinely?

Sara is a 6-year-old child who appears to have asthma and has a speech problem. She is seen by a community paediatrician. What type of information might be available about her?

Figure 2.1 sets out a probable history for Sara, as follows:

After birth Sara is registered (civil registration): this process counts the number of births locally and nationally.

An NHS number is created, and Sara is added to the local child health index and to a GP clinical system. The postcode will indicate in which lower super output area (LSOA) Sara resides, and the socioeconomic indicators related to that area should be available. (An LSOA is a small area for collating census data, consisting of about 600 households.)

Antenatal care information should record the smoking status of Sara's mother, maternal weight and other risk factors.

The birth record will have vital information about Sara, such as birth weight, and whether breastfeeding was initiated.

The health visitor's record, available electronically on the child health information system (CHIS), will record breastfeeding history, weight trajectory and developmental progress.

The GP record and the CHIS will record immunisation status – when immunised and what vaccine batch.

Sara attended Accident and Emergency (A&E) with wheezing – the attendance will be recorded, the date and time, and a diagnosis recorded.

Sara was admitted for an acute asthmatic episode – date of admission and of discharge and diagnosis on discharge are available electronically. Treatment is communicated to the GP by letter and added to the system.

The health visitor is concerned about developmental delay, particularly speech, and refers Sara to the speech therapist. The consultation is recorded but the outcome is not measured.

Sara attends the reception class at school and is weighed and measured. This data is recorded for the National Child Measurement Programme and shared with her parents and GP.

Sara has an assessment by the school nurse in order to develop a plan to manage her asthma. The consultation is recorded but the outcome is not measured. Figure 2.1 illustrates the collection of data in this case.

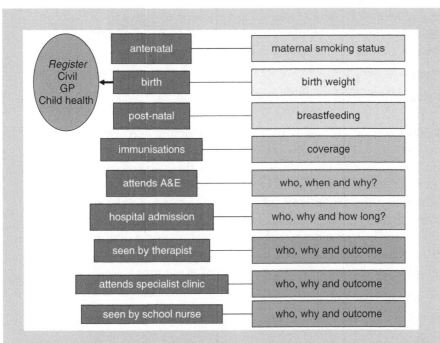

Figure 2.1 Routinely collected data in this example

So, returning to the community paediatrician, she could already have knowledge of the important demographic information, would probably have a complete record of attendances at A&E and would have the information on any admissions, and know the presumed diagnoses. However, the outcomes of each intervention are most likely to be parental- and child-reported rather than objective measures. The point of this is that most indicators are aggregates of measures or information held in a number of different ways by different agencies and collected by a wide range of individual professionals. This will have an impact on the quality of the data – and is discussed in more detail below.

How do we measure?

There are quantitative and qualitative methods for measuring relevant indicators and these have different strengths and weaknesses.

Quantitative methods

Quantitative information is information that can be counted or expressed numerically. Quantitative data can be presented visually in figures such as bar charts or tables. Much of the information provided in a joint strategic needs assessment is quantitative. Broadly, there are five ways of measuring: routine counts based on registration or notification processes, routine counts based on operational requirements, surveys, research studies and audits. These are not mutually exclusive.

Routine counts based on registration or notification processes

These may be mandatory on the professional or citizen (births, deaths, infectious diseases) or voluntary (reporting to a condition-specific surveillance centre, or claiming a social benefit). Usually a prescribed dataset is completed, the information is collated at an area or national level, and routine reports are produced at regular intervals. For example, the Office for National Statistics (ONS) is responsible for vital statistics (birth rates, mortality rates). New diagnoses of cancer are reported to the Cancer Intelligence Unit, which maintains records of individual cancer notification (previously known as regional cancer registries). Using postcodes allows the provision of aggregate data by age, gender, type, cancer site, stage and geographical area.

Routine counts based on operational requirements

These data are generated by an individual 'crossing a threshold' to attend or use a service. Attendances, admissions and contacts with a service are counted by organisations like hospitals to be able to quantify the business. One strong underlying reason for collecting numbers is financial, as income may be related to activity. (This is certainly true for NHS trusts providing acute hospital care as they are paid for a lot of what they do under the payment by results scheme.) However the data that are available do allow interrogation at various levels, and can be used to produce strategic information such as admission rates for selected conditions.

Surveys

Surveys are detailed studies gathering information about a population through observations and questionnaires. These are usually carried out on a sample but sometimes the whole target population is surveyed. The census is an example of a whole-population (strictly household) survey, whilst health surveys such as the English Health Survey are based on samples. Care is taken to make a sample as representative as possible, for example by sampling different strata.

Research studies

Epidemiological and other empirical studies can provide valuable information. They may be observational or experimental. Our understanding of the life course comes from longitudinal studies where a cohort is followed for many years and observations are made at different intervals. The Millennium cohort study, following children born in England in 2000, is a good example. Our understanding of risk factors is built on similar studies. Community surveys to ascertain the incidence and prevalence of a disease such as dementia are another example. These surveys use a standard case definition to determine the numbers of people with a particular condition.

Audits

An audit involves checking whether a standard is being applied or achieved in practice. In health terms this usually involves checking that a protocol or guideline for treatment is being met. For example, we know what level one blood marker (Hb1A) for good control of diabetes should be and the proportion of patients achieving that figure or less can be measured.

Qualitative methods

In public health work, qualitative data should be sought to complement the quantitative analysis. These types of data involve describing things in terms of categorisations or qualities. This will involve community engagement, and the process can, in itself, have a positive impact on health and wellbeing. Engaging with communities includes understanding whether services have delivered what was expected, and whether service users have had their needs met. Rapid participatory appraisal (see Chapter 3) is an approach that has the engagement of the community (often through community leaders) at its centre.

Qualitative data are gathered using a number of methods. These include ethno-anthropological methods such as focus groups, participant observation, interviews and surveys.

Focus groups

Focus groups are small groups selected from a wider population and sampled by open discussion for its members' opinions about a particular subject or area, and have been used especially in market research. The approach may be to explore pre-defined topics in a relatively structured way. Alternatively data are collected through unstructured discussion and treated as requiring analysis and interpretation. What participants say, along with aspects of interaction and group process, is examined for its connotation or meaning.

Participant observation

Participant observation refers to a form of sociological research methodology in which the researcher takes on a role in the social situation under observation. The researcher will become familiar with the key players and the community dynamics. The role is often described as either covert or overt. The aim is to experience events in the manner in which the subjects under study also experience these events. Participant observation is usually undertaken over an extended period of time, ranging from several months to many years. It is feasible for a community health worker to undertake this kind of research.

Interviews

Individual interviews may be structured or semistructured. A structured interview involves asking the respondent a list of predetermined questions about a specific topic. The interviewer may explain things the respondent does not understand. A semistructured interview will collect qualitative data by allowing a respondent the time and scope to talk about his or her opinions on a particular subject. The focus of the interview is decided beforehand and this determines the areas the interviewer wishes to explore. The objective is to understand the respondent's point of view rather than make generalisations. Usually the interviewer will use open-ended questions, e.g. Tell me about what you do to get physical exercise.

Surveys were mentioned above as one of the methods for gathering epidemiological data. Whereas a question such as 'How many units of alcohol do you drink each week?' will provide quantitative data, an open-ended question such as 'In what ways do you think drinking excess of alcohol is a problem?' will provide qualitative data.

Other methods for gathering information include citizens' juries, user and carer groups and deliberative polls.

Citizens' juries

These consist of a small panel of non-specialists, and are modelled on the functions of a criminal jury. The group sets out to examine the evidence relating to an issue of public significance in detail and delivers a 'verdict'.

User and carer groups

These groups have a special interest in and/or direct experience of a condition and can be approached as a focus group.

Deliberative polls

These measure what the public would think about a topic if they had adequate information to be able to reflect on the issues. Deliberative polling observes how the views of a citizen test group change as they learn more about the topic.

Postal or internet panels

These offer an alternative to seeking a new pool of potential respondents every time a survey is conducted. Internet panels may be self-selecting through a website or advertisement. Alternatively the panel can be created through invitation by random postal or telephone enquiry. The whole panel or a random selection can be surveyed about a topic, with or without sharing relevant information.

As stated above, the process can, in itself, have a positive impact on health and wellbeing. People and Participation.net, in describing what people can gain from participation, say:

> *Public participation is not only important for organisations in the public, private and not for profit sectors, it also has the potential to change how individuals and communities live and interact. Taking part in local decision-making or discussing future policy can have a transformative effect on how people think about themselves and their role in society.*
>
> (see People and Participation.net website, listed in references)

ACTIVITY 2.2

Look at Table 2.3. Think of an example when you would use each of the quantitative and qualitative methods to gather data, and complete the table.

Table 2.3 Quantitative and qualitative methods

Quantitative methods	Example of when you would use this method	Strengths and weaknesses
Routine counts based on registration/notification processes		
Routine counts based on operational requirements		
Surveys		
Research studies		
Audits		
Focus groups		
Participant observation		
Interviews		
Citizens' juries		
User and carer groups		
Deliberative polls		
Postal or internet panels		

Comment

Both quantitative and qualitative methods are used to gather data and for measuring relevant indicators. Each method has different strengths and weaknesses; choosing the right approach is what is important.

Quality of the data

The quality of the information is an important aspect of measuring to bear in mind continually. Three questions are important:

1. Where does the information actually come from?

2. How accurate and complete will the data be?

3. Are there any likely problems, such as potential for errors in collection, collation and interpretation (for example, through undersampling)?

The method of measuring will determine the quality of information available. In assessing the validity of an individual indicator there are a number of issues to consider. For example, the method of recording affects the accuracy of primary data source, whether written hard copy or real-time input into an electronic system. The method of data collection is important, for example, is it manual or electronic? Completeness and accuracy are affected by the number of times the data are copied or re-entered. Are the data collected as a routine task or not? If it is not a routine task it is subject to greater variation. If the data required come from multiple sources, consistency will be affected. Coding practice can vary; it is not a black and white process and some discretion may be used, which will lead to variation. Completeness of the data is often a problem. It means entering all the items every time. Finally, the timeliness of data entry will affect accuracy and retrospective collection or recording is more likely to lead to inaccuracy.

To assure data are complete, accurate and timely, it is helpful to have some kind of data quality process, usually known as data quality assurance.

What's the evidence?

The quality assurance project undertaken by the Information Services Division (ISD) of NHS Scotland assessed 34 data items from the maternity dataset (SMR02). They found that 18 (53 per cent) of the data items recorded on SMR02 matched the information found in the medical record/Scottish Woman-Held Maternity Record (SWHMR) in 90 per cent or more of the records, with eight data items matching 98 per cent and above.

Of the remaining 16 (47 per cent) data items that were recorded with less than 90 per cent of the records matching, five of these were very poorly recorded, with under 40 per cent matching. Recording these data items was optional at the time. As a result of the exercise it was recommended that four of the data items were made mandatory. The data items are:

1. typical weekly alcohol consumption;
2. drug misuse during this pregnancy;
3. ever injected illicit drugs;
4. drugs used.

The fifth poorly recorded data item was 'ethnic group'.

Four further data items that were poorly recorded, with 72–79 per cent of the records matching information in SWHMR, were:

1. height;
2. weight of mother at booking;
3. duration of labour;
4. analgesia during labour and/or delivery.

It seemed surprising that height and weight of mother at booking in particular should be recorded erroneously. Some hospital patient administration systems (PAS) are incorrectly rounding weight and 'duration of labour', which accounts for some of the differences.

For 'analgesia during labour and/or delivery', the most frequent unmatched record was where epidural had been recorded when information in medical records/ SWHMR showed the analgesia to be spinal. Also, analgesia was frequently recorded as unknown, none or left blank when SWHMR contained a specific analgesia.

Overall, in six of the 17 hospitals assessed, technical issues with the PAS either resulted in wrong information being extracted or data fields not allowing correct values to be entered. In approximately half of the hospitals assessed (eight hospitals), ISD found a small amount of patient documentation either missing or filed in the wrong patient record. The SWHMR was found to be structured and easy to use but completed to varying degrees across Scotland.

In addition, the requirement for some guidance was identified around the terminology used by midwives, and how medical records staff should interpret certain terms contained in SWHMR. Several definitional and clinical coding issues were identified throughout the assessment and these would be addressed by producing updated Coding Guidelines and revised training material, and offering training sessions to the hospital staff involved in SMR02 clinical coding.

(NHS National Services Scotland: Information Services Division, 2010)

Sources of data

There is a plethora of web-based data sources available to source indicators about health and wellbeing.

Mortality (death rates) and morbidity (prevalence and incidence, service use, disease management) for specific diseases/conditions can be found from a number of sources, such as the data held by the National Cancer Intelligence Network, the national register of congenital abnormalities and the mortality data published by the ONS. Health-related information such as indicators of deprivation and demographic data are derived from the National Census. Other sources of data include primary care settings, for example, GP registers, which are comprised of collated data accessed through the Quality Management and Analysis System (QMAS). The Quality and

IVERPOOL JOHN MOORES UNIVERSITY
LEARNING SERVICES

Outcomes Framework is another important source of data collected through the QMAS. Prescribing data is available by primary care trust (PCT). Sources of data from secondary care include hospital episodes (available from the Hospital Episode Statistics) and mental health data (including PCT-level mental health profiles).

The Compendium of Clinical and Health Indicators published in the Clinical and Health Outcomes Knowledge Base by the NHS Information Centre for health and social care is another useful source. Table 2.4 provides a summary of these different sources of data.

ACTIVITY 2.3

Look back at the measures we considered in Activity 2.1. Where is this indicator found and what quality issues need to be considered? Try and complete Table 2.5.

Table 2.5 Summary of sources of data

Measure	Source	Quality issues
Infant mortality		
Life expectancy		
Smoking		
Childhood obesity		
Alcohol admissions		
Accident mortality		
Hip fractures in elderly		
Suicide rate		
Dementia		
GCSE		
NEET		

NEET, not in education, employment or training.

Comment

Infant mortality, life expectancy, accident mortality, suicide rate and unemployment data are all available from the ONS. Infant mortality data are collated from data provided from regional maternity surveillance and are considered to be both complete and accurate. Life expectancy is an actuarial calculation based on age-specific mortality rates and the core data are complete and accurate. The accident mortality rate is complete and the accuracy rate is improved when coroners are involved. Similarly, the suicide rate is complete but accuracy is closely related to cultural interpretations as the coroner is involved, hence international comparisons may need caution. Unemployment rates are different to the claimant (jobseekers' allowance) count which, together with the inactive rate, balance the employed as 100 per cent of the 16–64-years population. Completeness and accuracy will depend on the definitions in use and comparisons, particularly when across different years, should take account of the eligibility criteria in place.

Table 2.4 Different sources of data

Dataset	Who provides it?	What does it include?
Population data		
Exeter System	Local NHS IT services	GP registrations of residents
ONS Mid-year Population Estimates	Office of National Statistics (ONS)	Population by area* one year in arrears
ONS Population Projections	ONS	District population data projected forward
Local Population Projections	ONS	Regional population data
Deaths		
Public Health Mortality Files	Local Government	All deaths occurring in area*
Annual Death Registrations Extract	Local Government	All deaths registered in area*
Births and Maternity data		
Public Health Birth Files	ONS	All births to area* residents
Annual Births extract	ONS	All births to area* residents
Congenital anomalies	ONS	Congenital anomalies recorded at birth
Breast feeding	Local NHS IT Services	Feeding regime initiated at birth
Vaccination and Immunisations	NHS Child Health Dept/Health Protection Agency	Vaccine uptake for MMR, whooping cough
Teenage (U18) Conceptions	Dept for Education (DfE)	U18 conceptions by district
Terminations	Dept for Education (DfE) ONS	Variable data on terminations at area* level
Hospital Activity		
XIOM database/data warehouse	Local NHS IT services	Multi-facet NHS data
Local Provider database	Local NHS IT services	Multi-facet NHS data
Community Data		
Breast screening	PCT/LCG/screening programme level	Screening invitation uptake
Cervical Screening	PCT/LCG/screening programme level	Screening invitation uptake
Mental Health Community System	Local NHS IT services	Contacts with Community Mental Health professionals
Smoking Cessation	Local Smoking Advisory Service	Smoking quitters
Cancer data - registrations, survival rates, etc.	PHOs/Cancer intelligence service	All cancer cases registered in area*
Sexual Health Clinic data	Health Protection Agency	Referrals by specific diagnosis
Prescribing	EPACT system	Practice prescribing data

Dataset	Who provides it?	What does it include?
Socio-economic data		
Census 2001	ONS	Tabulations of census questions responses
Neighbourhood Statistics & MAIDeN	ONS	Multi-agency data at Lower Layer Super Output Area level (LSOA) & small area level
Deprivation		
Indices of Deprivation (2004)	Dept for Communities & Local Government	Calculated deprivation scores at LSOA level
Health Poverty	NHS Information Centre for Health & Social Care	Calculated index scores at district level
Index Fuel poverty	Centre for Sustainable Energy website	Calculated index scores at Lower LSOA level
Lifestyle Data		
Health and Lifestyle Survey	Local PCT/LCG	Survey results from questionnaire (topics vary)
Health Survey for England	ONS	Survey results from questionnaire (topics vary)
Key Public Health Data Publications		
Compendium of Clinical & Health Indicators	Dept of Health/NCHOD	Multi-indicator data at PCO, district, regional & national levels
Vital Statistics (VS) data	ONS	Births and deaths
Area profiles	Audit commission/APHO	Multi-indicator health summary at district, borough and county level
Reference		
International Classification of Diseases versions 9/10	World Health Organisation	Disease classification
National Administrative Codes Service (NACS)	NHS Connecting for health	Codes and lookups for NHS management

* This could be at county and district or county council/London Borough/Unitary Authority level or regional level

APHO – Association of Public Health Observatories
LGC – Local Commissioning Group
NCHOD – National Centre for Health Outcomes Development
PCT – Primary Care Trust
PHOs – Public Health Observatories

Alcohol admission and the number of hip fractures are collected through Hospital Episode Statistics and both are dependent upon the coding practice in hospital and the completeness and accuracy of the clinical record.

Childhood obesity, measured through the National Child Measurement Programme, is considered to be of good quality as a high percentage of children are measured, although the data are not complete. Smoking prevalence, on the other hand, is based on self-reported data that are extrapolated to provide local estimates. The validity is not checked so as such these data are of poorer quality; however, these are the best available data.

The percentage of students achieving 5 A*–C results, including English and maths, and the percentage of young people aged 16–18 not in education, employment or training (NEET) are both available from the Department for Education website, **www.education.gov.uk**. The GCSE rate is complete and accurate while the NEET rate is dependent upon local notifications.

It is important when considering the range of available health-related indicators to consider the source of the data and the completeness and accuracy. Chapter 4 considers the quality of information in more detail.

Chapter summary

In this chapter we have discussed the features of different measures used to describe health and wellbeing, and identified the key issues to consider in using these measures or indicators. This will enable you to take a critical approach to selecting indicators to use when undertaking a health needs assessment discussed in Chapter 3.

GOING FURTHER

APHO (2008) *The Good Indicators Guide: Understanding How to Use and Choose Indicators*. London: NHS Institute for Innovation and Improvement.
This guide is intended to be a short, practical resource for anyone who is responsible for using indicators to monitor and improve performance, systems or outcomes. It aims to balance what is desirable in terms of using indicators in the most rigorous way with what is practical and achievable in healthcare settings.

Hashagen, S (2003) Framework for measuring community health and wellbeing (Chapter 17), in Orme, J, Powell, J, Taylor, P, Harrison, T and Grey, M (eds) (2003) *Public Health for the 21st Century: New Perspectives on Policy, Participation and Practice*. Maidenhead: McGraw-Hill/Open University Press.
This chapter is a useful mix of theory and practical advice for measuring aspects of health and wellbeing at a community level.

chapter 3

Doing a Health Needs Assessment

Mike Lavender

Meeting the Public Health Competences

This chapter will help you to evidence the following competences for public health (Public Health Skills and Career Framework):

- Level 5(1): Collect and collate routine data on health and wellbeing and needs using a range of tools and techniques;
- Level 6(c): Understanding of strengths, uses, interpretation and limitations of various types of data relating to health and wellbeing, needs and outcomes;
- Level 6(d): Understanding of links between, and relative importance of, the various determinants of health and wellbeing and needs;
- Level 6(e): Understanding of the concept and nature of inequalities in health and wellbeing (including use of social deprivation indices);
- Level 7(1): Assess and describe the health and wellbeing and needs of specific populations and the inequities in health and wellbeing experienced by populations, communities and groups;
- Level 7(6): Interpret and apply indicators for monitoring the population's health and wellbeing;
- Level 7(a) Understanding of qualitative and quantitative sources and methods for measuring, analysing and interpreting health and wellbeing, needs and outcomes;
- Level 8(2): Assess and describe the health and wellbeing and needs of populations using a variety of methods.

This chapter will also assist you in demonstrating the following National Occupational Standards for public health:

- Advise others on data and information related to health and wellbeing and/or stressors to health and wellbeing and its uses (PHP08);
- Collect and link data and information about the health and wellbeing and related needs of a defined population (PHP10);
- Analyse and interpret data and information about the health and wellbeing and related needs of a defined population (PHP11).

This chapter will also be useful in demonstrating Standard 6 of the Public Health Practitioner Standards.

Standard 6

Obtain, verify, analyse and interpret data and/or information to improve the health and wellbeing outcomes of a population/community/group – demonstrating:

a. knowledge of the importance of accurate and reliable data/information and the anomalies that might occur;
b. knowledge of the main terms and concepts used in epidemiology and the routinely used methods for analysing quantitative and qualitative data;
c. ability to make valid interpretations of the data and/or information and communicate these clearly to a variety of audiences.

Overview

This chapter explores the concept of health needs assessments (HNA) as a means of identifying and prioritising the health needs of a community or population group and will help you to consider the implications for improving health and wellbeing. It will also help you to develop your thinking about the nature of health, need and HNA. In this chapter we will consider different types of need, such as expressed need, met need, comparative need and felt need, and the relationship between these and demand and supply. We will also consider different approaches to HNAs described in the literature and look at contemporary frameworks used in the literature to explain how to carry out and conduct an HNA. The chapter goes on to set out different approaches to carrying out an HNA, in particular the two-stage (epidemiological) approach and a commonly used five-step method. The final section of the chapter discusses two tools (rapid participatory appraisal and problem tree analysis) for increasing community involvement in HNA.

Exercises in this chapter will focus on:

• the use of health profiles in identifying health needs;
• ways to estimate health need and, in particular, unmet need;
• key questions to be considered and addressed when conducting an HNA;
• using rapid participatory appraisal in HNA.

This chapter uses theory, tools and case studies to explore the nature of health, need and HNA.

After reading this chapter you will be able to:

• discuss concepts of health and need;
• define and describe what an HNA is and how it can be used to improve health and wellbeing;
• describe the range of approaches that currently influence thinking and practice underpinning HNAs;
• understand how to plan and carry out an HNA;
• articulate the range of options available for undertaking an HNA and for ensuring you choose the most appropriate approach for your task.

Health, health needs and health needs assessment

In most cases an HNA is carried out by a team, so it is important that there is shared agreement and a common language for the terms used. For example, the team will need to have a common understanding about what it is they are assessing – in particular what they mean by 'health' and what they mean by 'need'.

What do we mean by 'health'?

Health is defined in a number of ways, ranging from the absence of disease (Scadding, 1988, p123) to a more positive concept that emphasises social and personal resources, as well as physical capabilities. The World Health Organization's definition of health as *a state of complete physical, psychological, and social wellbeing and not simply the absence of disease or infirmity* (WHO, 1948) remains the most enduring. While this definition has been criticised for being unachievable, for rendering the majority of the population as being unhealthy (as it ignores human capacity to adapt to physical, emotional and social challenges and ability to achieve a sense of wellbeing with chronic disease or disability) and for being difficult to operationalise (Huber *et al.*, 2011) it does embrace a social model of health which views health and well-being as a consequence of wider determinants of health (see discussion in Chapter 1).

What do we mean by 'need'?

Bradshaw's taxonomy of need is a helpful starting point (Bradshaw, 1972). Normative need is a need identified according to a norm (or set standard) generally set by professionals. Comparative need concerns problems which emerge through comparison with others who are not in need. One of the most common uses of this approach has been the comparison of social problems in different areas in order to determine which areas are most deprived. Felt need is need which people feel and is therefore a need that is based on the perspective of those who have the need.

Expressed need is the need that people say they have. People can feel need which they do not express and, similarly, needs can be expressed that are not felt needs. These different categories of need are summarised in Table 3.1.

Table 3.1 Bradshaw's categorisation of need

Felt need	Individual perception of variation from normal health
Expressed need	Individual seeks help to overcome variation from normal health
Normative need	Professionally defined intervention appropriate for the expressed need
Comparative need	Comparison between needs of different groups

It is also important to distinguish between need, demand and supply. In the context of healthcare needs assessment, Stevens and Raftery (1994) define need, demand and supply in an approach that includes important health economic principles:

- Need is the population's ability to benefit from health (and social) care interventions.

- Demand is what people would be willing to pay for in a market or might wish to use in a system of free healthcare.

- Supply is what is provided and this will be determined by political and policy priorities and available resources.

Demand for services is the expression of felt need and is influenced by a range of factors, including illness behaviour, the media and the supply of and knowledge of services. There is a direct relationship between the supply and accessibility of services and demand. Figure 3.1 shows the relationship between felt need and demand (or expressed need) and professionally defined need (or normative need). Identifying the unmet need, i.e. the extent to which professionally defined need is not met by the supply of current services, is a key element of an HNA. Unmet need is then a priority for service change to ensure greater alignment between supply and professionally defined need.

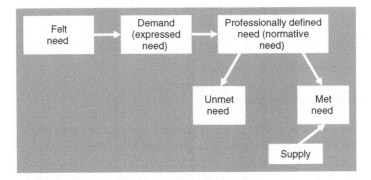

Figure 3.1 Relationship between need, demand and supply

What do we mean by health needs assessment?

HNA is *a systematic method of identifying the health and healthcare needs of a population and making recommendations for changes to meet these needs* (Wright *et al.*, 1998, p1310). Hooper and Longworth (2002, p3) define HNA as a *systematic and explicit process, which reviews the health issues affecting a population* and *aims to improve health, and reduce health inequalities, by identifying local priorities for change and then planning the actions needed to make these changes happen*. Cavanagh and Chadwick (2005, p3) likewise define HNA as *a systematic method for reviewing the health issues facing a population, leading to agreed priorities and resource allocation that will improve health and reduce inequalities*. Thus HNAs provide a systematic approach to the reduction of inequalities in health and informing the decision-making and change management processes to improve health.

A number of different approaches to developing an HNA have been described in the literature (Stevens and Raftery, 1994; Wright *et al.*, 1998; Wright, 2001; Hooper and Longworth, 2002; Cavanagh and Chadwick, 2005). Stevens and Raftery (1994) distinguish between epidemiological, comparative and corporate HNA (see Figure 3.2).

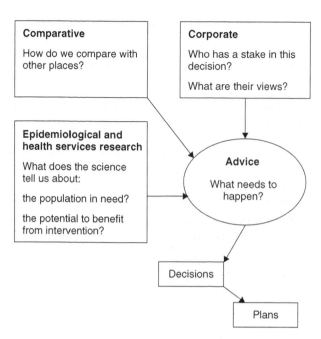

Figure 3.2 Health needs assessment perspectives

Source: Elkheir (2007) (reproduced with permission).

Epidemiological health needs assessment

Epidemiological health needs assessment begins with a consideration of the population in need and the potential to benefit from an intervention. This approach uses largely quantitative data and the focus is on prevalence, incidence, service provision between different populations and evidence of effective interventions. It is less concerned with community perspectives on the health topic, focusing as it does primarily on healthcare needs.

Comparative health needs assessment

This approach involves comparing the experience of poor health among one group with another, often by focusing on services in one area with another. Variations in cost and service activity adjusted for the different populations (standardisation) generate questions about service provision. A good source of information for this approach is the NHS Comparators website (**www.ic.nhs.uk/nhscomparators**). NHS Comparators is an analytical service for commissioners and providers. It helps improve the quality of care delivered by benchmarking and comparing activity and costs on a local, regional and national level.

Corporate health needs assessment

A corporate HNA may use both epidemiological and comparative data but also considers the perspectives of key stakeholders and is a synthesis of the views from interested parties, including professional, public and patient views. This approach can provide important local information (i.e. community engagement and user involvement) that complements other available information.

All three approaches provide some indication on what needs to happen, which in turn should lead to decisions on actions and an action plan that can feed into the planning cycle to deliver proposed changes. Whichever approach is chosen there is a need to involve local communities, services users and the public in need assessment. The draft guidance on JSNAs referred to in Chapter 1 (DoH, 2012) envisages insights from communities being used alongside other evidence to inform decisions, with an emphasis on tackling the wider determinants of health. The guidance sees a two-way street of communication in which users and the public are helped to understand the factors that influence services in their area and they in turn have the opportunity to shape those services.

Health needs assessment and the planning cycle

HNA in a range of different forms has always been a core part of healthcare planning. However, HNAs took on a more central role following the public sector reforms of the 1990s in which the concept of commissioning was introduced. The essential role of commissioners is to use the resources available to achieve optimum gain in health and wellbeing by providing for the needs of the population that has been prioritised. This is carried out in the wider context of rising healthcare costs, the introduction of new technology and treatments, a rising demand for health and care due to an increasingly older population and improved survival following heart attacks and strokes, and an increase in public expectation driven partly by an increased political emphasis on greater patient choice. These are demand-related issues and are key challenges facing those who commission services. On the supply side, commissioners have to make some difficult choices. These include judgements on the effectiveness, appropriateness and quality of services in the context of limited resources and inequities in healthcare provision. HNAs can help to alleviate the challenges of the decision-making process by providing a robust framework for systematically assessing all the relevant information about the health of a population, enabling community, public and patient involvement in the process and identifying the gaps in data, information or local knowledge that are needed before making decisions about services. HNAs should therefore be central to the decision-making process for identifying priorities and improving services, as illustrated in Figure 3.3.

Preliminary questions to consider before carrying out an HNA

An HNA needs time, resources and a clear focus to be effective. It also requires a number of key questions to be addressed prior to starting work on data collection to ensure that the HNA provides information to help decision makers decide on health priorities and to provide a basis for the HNA project plan. The following eight questions can provide a useful indication of the level of resource and how much time will be needed.

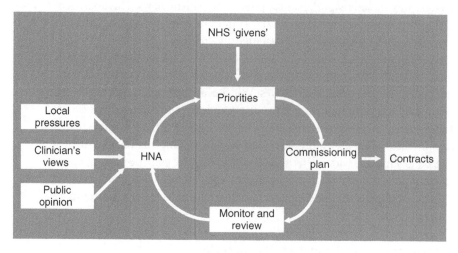

Figure 3.3 Health needs assessment (HNA) and the planning cycle

What is the background to the HNA?

It is useful to know the reason why the HNA is being carried out. For example, is there a specific problem that has prompted the call for an HNA?

What is the population (or patient group) to be assessed?

The size of the population under consideration, or the prevalence and impact of a condition experienced by a patient group, will determine the scale of the HNA. For example, is the HNA aimed at the level of a general practitioner (GP) practice population or will it cover a wider area? An HNA for a relatively uncommon condition (such as end-stage renal failure) should only be carried out at a regional level with a population in millions, whereas for common conditions (such as type 2 diabetes), an HNA at a GP practice level is feasible. Figure 3.4 illustrates this.

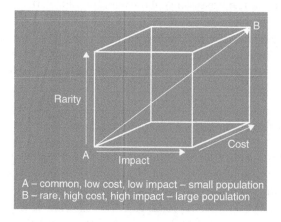

Figure 3.4 Population suitable for health needs assessment (HNA)

Source: Wright *et al.* (1998) (reproduced with permission).

What is the question being asked?

The focus of an HNA should be clear about the distinction between:

- the need for health and the need for healthcare;
- the need for healthcare services and the need for other services (e.g. social care);
- individual need and population need.

Who wants to know the answer?

An HNA is part of a decision-making process for identifying health priorities and doing something about them to improve health and service provision. Are the people who have asked for the HNA part of that decision-making process? Will they act on the findings of the HNA and do they have the authority and control of the necessary resources to make decisions?

What are the expectations of those involved?

Unless you are working on the HNA alone (which is highly unlikely), others will be involved. Do all of the contributors have a common understanding of what the HNA is about and what can realistically be achieved?

What resources are available for the HNA and what is the timescale?

HNA needs time to be done properly so it is important to ensure that there is sufficient time set aside to work on the HNA. Will you have support of others in the team, such as data analysts? Do you have a budget for community venues, postal surveys and focus groups?

What work has already been carried out?

A good starting point is to find out whether an HNA has already been carried out. The Director of Public Health's Annual Report is usually a good source of health profiles and topic-specific needs assessments. Joint strategic needs assessments will provide a useful overview of the population at a local-authority level and an HNA carried out in another area may also be useful. Taking the findings from elsewhere and applying them to the local population after making suitable adjustments for age, gender and socioeconomic characteristics will give you a good idea of the size of the problem that can be refined with more local data. The Health Care Needs Assessment website contains a number of useful topic-specific assessments (see the Going Further section at the end of the chapter).

Are the key stakeholders signed up to the HNA project?

The way to ensure the support of all key stakeholders is to prepare a project plan for the HNA that includes the aims and objectives of the project, the resources needed, the format and content of the final report and the timescale in which the project should be completed.

Having reviewed the answers to these questions and decided that there is a need to carry out an HNA, there are a number of approaches that can be used. Two commonly used approaches are the two-stage approach and the five-step approach and elements of each are frequently described in the literature. Other approaches referred to as developmental approaches attempt to increase community engagement in the process. Rapid participatory appraisal and problem tree analysis are two techniques that are utilised to engage local communities in the HNA process. These different approaches are described in the following section.

A two-stage framework for carrying out an HNA

One approach to conducting an HNA is to break it down into two distinct but related stages: stage 1, health profiling and identifying priorities and stage 2, indepth assessment of a health priority. Stage 1 includes gathering all the relevant information that describes the health of the defined population and using predetermined criteria for selecting health priorities for more indepth analysis. Stage 2 involves a systematic review of all the relevant information about the need, demand and supply for the selected health priority. Figure 3.5 shows the relationship between these two stages.

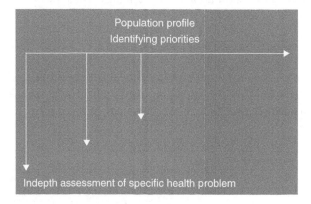

Figure 3.5 Health profiling and indepth assessment of priorities

Stage 1: Health profiling and identifying priorities

This stage of the HNA process is about gathering the information that describes the overall health of the target population and is based on guidelines for undertaking an HNA (Hooper and Longworth, 2002).

Population

How many people are in the target population? A useful way of grouping this information is under the headings of person, place and time.

- person: age, gender, socioeconomic status, ethnicity;
- place: where they live, the characteristics of the area, environmental factors;

- time: any recent changes in the population such as new housing developments, trends in employment.

Health indicators

Collect information from routine data sources that describe the overall health of the target population such as:

- standardised death rates – all cause and for the major causes of death such as cardiovascular disease and cancer;

- prevalence of long-term conditions on GP practice registers and self-reported long-term disability from the census;

- prevalence of determinants of health such as smoking, blood pressure and obesity.

Service utilisation

This could include indicators such as immunisation coverage, uptake of screening programmes, the use of hospital services, quit rates with the stop smoking service.

The most reliable and consistent sources of routine data (which were referred to in Chapter 2) include:

- Compendium of Clinical Indicators;

- hospital activity data;

- census information;

- GP practice data.

In addition there may be local surveys or audits, which have reliable information about local services.

Choosing priorities

This is arguably the most difficult step in the HNA process. Any conclusions at this stage could be challenged as being biased or incorrect. There are steps you can take that will get over these challenges. For example, ensuring that the information gathered is as complete as possible, ignoring or excluding any information not directly relevant to the aims and objectives of the HNA, being selective in the information you use to select priorities and having clear criteria for the decisions made can mitigate against such challenges. The criteria for selecting priorities should be agreed in advance. For example, the selection criteria could include:

- the size of the problem;

- the effectiveness of any interventions;

- the acceptability and feasibility of making any changes;

- public, user and carer views;

- the resources needed for any change;
- the degree of influence and control the key stakeholders have over the priorities selected.

Health profiling provides an overview but much of the information needed to select priorities can only be gathered by a more indepth assessment in stage 2. By involving stakeholders at the profiling stage a consensus on priorities based on the available information can be reached prior to going on to the next stage.

ACTIVITY 3.1

Get copies of your local Director of Public Health's Annual Report and the joint strategic needs assessment from your local authority.

Using the information in these reports create a health profile for your area.

What are the biggest health problems in the local community?

How do these compare with regional or national levels?

What are the possible explanations for any differences?

Do the Annual Report and the JSNA identify the priorities clearly? What criteria were used to prioritise? Using the criteria above, do you come to the same conclusions?

Comment

The DPH Annual Report and the JSNA will contain core information in line with the core dataset. A profile equivalent to (or copy of) the local health profiles produced by the APHO may be included in one or both. Use this after you have created a profile to compare the items you have selected to put in the profile. In a typical population in the UK, the trend towards an older population, the prevalence of long-term conditions, the large contribution of CVD and cancers to death rates, and inequalities will be obvious findings.

Your explanations for the differences with national rates should reflect your understanding of the wider determinants of health (which were discussed in Chapter 1), and how they influence health and wellbeing locally.

Your priorities and those identified by the reports should be similar using the available data, unless there has been a strong component of listening to the community when there may be some surprises!

Stage 2: Indepth assessment of a health priority

This stage concerns the indepth assessment of a specific health priority for action and is often referred to as *epidemiological needs assessment*. This health priority may have been identified through the stage 1 health profiling or in some other way.

The objective of this stage is to gather all the relevant information about the health priority. Often this stage is a combination of epidemiology, health economics and service review and informed by Epidemiologically Based Needs Assessment protocols that are typically used in healthcare needs assessments. There are three components of this approach: the size of the problem, effectiveness and cost-effectiveness of interventions and provision of current services.

Size of the problem

This is an assessment of the incidence and prevalence of the disease, to determine how many people will need the service or intervention. Incidence and prevalence are defined in Chapter 1.

Effectiveness and cost-effectiveness of interventions

This is an assessment of the benefit of the service or intervention and at what cost.

Provision of current services

This involves carrying out a baseline assessment of current services to identify the gaps and possible opportunities to disinvest in order to fill these gaps.

The triangulation of these three components will provide stakeholders with a comprehensive epidemiological view of the health priority.

Case Study: Assessing the 'unmet need' for chronic obstructive pulmonary disease

The British Lung Foundation published a report entitled *Invisible Lives: Chronic Obstructive Pulmonary Disease (COPD) – Finding the Missing Millions* (British Lung Foundation, 2007). It states that there are an estimated 3.7 million people with COPD in the UK, yet only 900,000 people have been diagnosed. This means there are an estimated 2.8 million people who have undiagnosed COPD; if left untreated, this illness could severely restrict their lives and eventually kill them. The report authors used the Mosaic lifestyle segmentation matched with the area of residence of people admitted to hospital with COPD to predict risk of future hospital admission by lifestyle type. The different levels of risk could then be applied to different populations to estimate future admission rates. The report shows that NHS Ayrshire and Arran is ranked 18th out of 192 primary care organisations in the UK, with a 37 per cent higher risk of future hospital admission with COPD than the UK average.

The authors wanted to know how the number of patients registered with general practices in Ayrshire and Arran on the COPD Quality and Outcomes Framework (QOF) registers compared with the expected number of patients. (The QOF is a component of the General Medical Services contract for general practices, and practices earn points for different items, including adding patients to disease-specific registers.)

The COPD Prevalence Modeller is provided by the Eastern Region Public Health Observatory (Nacul et al., 2007) and is based on the Health Survey for England 2001. This was a survey of a representative sample of the population of England who had lung function tests and data collected on relevant risk factors. The model takes account of gender, age, smoking status, ethnicity, area of residence and an area-based index of deprivation.

The COPD Prevalence Model estimates a prevalence of 4.3 per cent for people aged 15 years and above registered with practices in Ayrshire and Arran. This means that there are an estimated 14,587 people with COPD. The actual number of people with COPD on practice QOF registers in 2008–09 was 8,528, which is 58 per cent of the estimated total. This means that there are approximately 6,000 people in Ayrshire and Arran who have undiagnosed COPD. There is no discernible relationship between the actual and estimated prevalence at practice level, suggesting that the variation in the QOF-registered prevalence has more to do with practice characteristics than with underlying need.

ACTIVITY 3.2

Looking at the COPD prevalence in Ayrshire and Arran – the 'missing thousands' case study and the different types of 'need' outlined in Figure 3.1 – identify the estimates for each type of need for the population of Ayrshire and Arran in respect of COPD.

- How were the estimates of numbers derived? What factors will affect the accuracy of those numbers?
- What explanations are there for the amount of unmet need?
- What methods could you propose to assess this need?

Comment

The box labelled unmet need will show approximately 6,000 people with COPD who are unknown to primary care, or who have COPD but do not have a diagnosis of COPD recorded.

The estimate of the numbers with COPD in the population is made by applying the rate determined through the results of the Health Survey for England. The case definition of COPD was defined including the results of spirometry (a lung function test) using joint American Thoracic Society and European Respiratory Society criteria. If the cases were defined through self-reported respiratory symptoms alone, then the validity of the rate derived from the survey would be questionable. The sample size of the survey may mean the confidence intervals for the rates by level of deprivation are wide. The smoking rates are probably synthetic (estimates). So the model used to estimate numbers might have a wide range for any given area.

The accuracy of QOF numbers depends on factors such as the willingness to give a diagnosis or a 'label' to the patient and recording it in a consistent way so it is picked up through the coding system. Patients with COPD may be under treatment but without the formal diagnosis.

The unmet need may be real or simply predicted. The best way to assess this would be to do a community survey with a large enough sample, using a clear case definition and an objective clinical test such as spirometry.

Protocol for the epidemiological approach to HNA

Stevens and Raftery (1994) set out a protocol for conducting an epidemiological HNA structured under the following headings:

Statement of the problem

A precise statement of the problem and its context makes it clear what is to be assessed in terms of need and what is outside the scope of the exercise. Often this will be influenced by the major priorities relevant to healthcare commissioners.

Subcategories

This is about subdividing a diseases-specific population group, for example by severity or prognosis. In the context of healthcare needs assessment, what is most useful to a commissioner is a subcategorisation that is predictive of requirements for services.

Prevalence and incidence

The frequency of occurrence of disease is a core part of the epidemiological approach to needs assessment. Prevalence is most useful in healthcare needs assessment when it can be directly related to the subdivision (say, severity of disease) that predicts service requirements.

Services available

Information about structure (e.g. how many doctors specialising in the condition per unit of population) and process (how many people attend a service per unit of population) is relevant to this section.

Effectiveness and cost-effectiveness

Effectiveness and cost-effectiveness were defined in Chapter 1. The information on these aspects of an intervention or service has improved dramatically in recent years. There is now a commonly used system for grading the benefit and the strength of evidence for interventions.

Models of care

A flexible approach is needed to models of care based on need. Sometimes these-models are based on four tiers of service from self-management to highly specialised care, or on a care pathway from prevention to end-of-life care. Lack of agreement on thresholds for intervention is often an issue. For example, should cataract operations be offered at a given level of (poor) visual acuity, or based on the impact on the patient's life?

Outcomes and targets

The principal objective of healthcare needs assessment is the specification of services and other activities that impinge upon healthcare. Increasingly there is an emphasis on defining the desired outcomes from those activities, which include clinical improvement and patient/carer experience. Outcomes are discussed in Chapter 5.

A five-step approach to HNA

Other approaches to needs assessment include Hooper and Longworth's (2002) and Cavanagh and Chadwick's (2005) five-step approach, as illustrated in Figure 3.6. This is similar to the step approach to project planning described in Chapter 8 of the *Leading for Health and Wellbeing* book in this series.

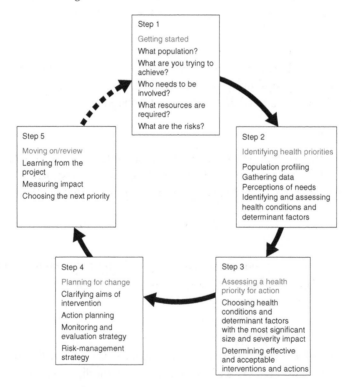

Figure 3.6 The five-step approach

Step 1: Getting started

In this first step the aim is to define clearly the population that will be the focus of the HNA and to provide a rationale for choosing this population. Being clear about why the population has been chosen, what you are trying to achieve, who needs to be involved, obtaining the resources that are needed, anticipating and dealing with potential challenges and constraints and minimising risks and ensuring that the project stays on track are important elements of this step. As Cavanagh and Chadwick (2005, p9) note, HNAs *are worthwhile undertaking only if they result in changes that will benefit the population. It is therefore essential to be realistic and honest about what you are capable of achieving* so being realistic about what can be achieved is critical.

Step 2: Identifying health priorities

Having undertaken the first step, the population should now be clear and the challenge in this step is to identify health priorities for the population. Developing a profile of the health of this population, gathering data and perceptions of need in order to identify priorities is the key focus of this step. Consideration should be given in this stage to methods that involve the population, such as focus groups, interviews, questionnaires and other developmental approaches to HNAs to increase engagement in the decision-making process. Once health priorities have been identified, Cavanagh and Chadwick (2005) suggest using 'impact' and 'changeability' (where you ask *can the most significant health conditions and determinant factors be changed effectively by those involved in the assessment?*) as criteria for selecting health priorities for action.

Step 3: Assessing a health priority for action

In step 3 'acceptability' and 'resource feasibility' are two further selection criteria that can be used. Cavanagh and Chadwick (2005, p35) propose revisiting steps 1 and 2 and then applying these criteria. Identifying acceptable changes for this health priority involves being clear about whether interventions would be acceptable to the target population group as well as the wider community and to those who might be delivering the intervention. Organisations commissioning and/or providing the activity will also need to find proposed interventions acceptable. The resource implications of the proposed interventions also need to be considered and perceived as feasible. Questions such as whether existing resources can be used differently, what actions will achieve the greatest impact on health for the resources used and how resource needs can be met are important in assessing priorities for action.

Step 4: Planning for change

This step concentrates on how to implement the changes and set out clear aims and objectives together with actions to achieve these. The priority areas identified in the previous step should form the basis for action planning. Being clear about what actions are required and who will take responsibility for each of these areas and within what timeframes are key elements to be agreed in this step. Agreeing key milestones and the processes that will be put in place for monitoring and evaluation are essential to ensure that the actions are monitored. Most approaches to HNA make a distinction between process and outcome measures that form part of the evaluation of the success of an HNA. Agreeing and recording an action plan is therefore an

Table 3.2 Key parameters in an action plan

Health priority actions	Who will take this forward?	In what timescale?	How?	Progress to date
Example: To provide home safety equipment for teenage parents with children aged under five	Primary care trust Young parents lead Health visitor Children's centre family liaison worker	All teenage parents to have received information and support by April 2013	Home safety equipment to be available through home safety loan scheme	Young parents lead, health visitor working with teenage parents and family liaison worker all participated in project plan, clear about roles and links with one another

important aspect of this step. Table 3.2 provides an illustration of key parameters that should form part of the monitoring of an action plan.

An additional focus in this step is to manage potential risks to delivering the changes identified. Cavanagh and Chadwick (2005) and Hooper and Longworth (2002) stress the importance of incorporating a risk management strategy throughout the HNA.

Step 5: Moving on and review

This final step provides an opportunity to reflect on the HNA process and involves consideration of what went well and why. Identifying further action and considering main challenges are all useful ways to learn from the HNA. Improvement in health conditions and status following the interventions should also be captured.

ACTIVITY 3.3

Think of an area that could usefully be the focus of an HNA in your area. Now work through each of the five steps described and identify the key questions you would need to answer in each of these steps.

Comment

You may have found it relatively straightforward to identify key questions that need to be addressed. Often the challenge is in getting agreement and consensus among those who are involved in the HNA. Table 3.3 summarises key questions that should be considered and addressed in each of these five steps. You might like to reflect both on the areas that you identified and those that you did not think of.

Table 3.3 Key questions in the five-step approach

Step	Key questions to be considered and addressed in each step
Step 1	Who is the population? Why has this population been chosen? What are you trying to achieve? What are the aims and specific objectives? Who needs to be involved? Who has a stake in this health needs assessment (HNA)? What resources will be needed? What challenges and constraints might there be and how can these risks be minimised? How will you ensure the project stays on track?
Step 2	How many people are in the target group? Where are they located? What data are currently available about the population? What are the main common experiences and differences within the group? How does the population perceive its needs? What factors determine the health status? How does the determinant factor affect health? What is the impact on health? Which of the priority health conditions/determinant factors can be effectively improved by those involved? Are these local and national priorities? To what extent does choosing these health priorities help to reduce health inequalities? Have you shared these findings with the key stakeholders? Have you engaged them in decision making?
Step 3	Who is being assessed by whom and why? What is the aim of the HNA? What are the boundaries? Have determinant factors been identified? What are the factors that are likely to have the most significant impact? Changeability? What interventions were considered most effective and acceptable? What are the resource implications and are these feasible?
Step 4	What are the aims and objectives? What actions are required and who will take responsibility for each of these areas? In what timescales? What processes will be put in place for monitoring and evaluation? What will be the key indicators of success? What outcome measures will be used? What are the risks in taking these changes forward?
Step 5	What was achieved by the project? How did it contribute to reducing inequalities? What needs to happen next? What new priority was chosen for the population? What main message from the last HNA will you take forward to the next?

Source: Adapted from Hooper and Longworth (2002) and Cavanagh and Chadwick (2005).

Developmental approaches to HNA: tools for increasing community involvement

A common (and often justified) criticism of many HNAs is the lack of follow-through into project plans, commissioning decisions or service developments. There are some approaches to needs assessment that aim to bridge the gap between analysis and action.

In the UK the inclusion of public and patient views in HNA has been variable and limited in scope. There are some exceptions and experience has shown that when the public are directly involved in need assessment and service planning, the results are more likely to lead to changes that reflect the needs of the community (Popay *et al.*, 2007, pp43–49). Over the last two decades rural and urban development programmes have used more participatory approaches to identifying health needs and planning new projects to the extent that in some areas these approaches have become the norm. Participatory appraisal (often referred to as rapid participatory appraisal) and problem tree analysis are techniques that can be used to encourage community participation and involvement in HNA. Participation in an HNA can range from being a source of information, providing a community perspective on perceptions of need to more influential approaches that identify needs and determine how these should be prioritised.

Rapid participatory appraisal

Rapid participatory appraisal methods aim to involve people and communities actively in identifying problems, formulating plans and implementing decisions. This approach is a type of corporate needs assessment that is explicitly aimed at gaining the perspectives of the community that will benefit from any services being planned. Rapid participatory appraisal methods seek to gain community perspectives of local health and social needs and to incorporate these findings into plans for service developments. Such methods have been designed to gather relevant information in a limited period of time to ensure that they contribute to any planning decisions and are underpinned by principles of equity, participation and collaboration. Data are collected generally from three main sources (Murray, 1999, p441):

1. interviews with a range of local informants;

2. existing written records about the neighbourhood;

3. observations made in the neighbourhood or in the homes of the interviewees.

Murray (1999, p441) suggests that this information can be used to form an 'information pyramid' that describes the problems and priorities in the neighbourhood, that has a foundation based on strong community information, as illustrated in Figure 3.7.

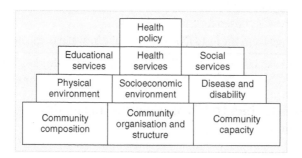

Figure 3.7 Information pyramid used in rapid participatory appraisal

Source: Murray (1999, p441) (reproduced with permission).

Data collected from one source are validated by checking with data from at least two other sources or methods of collection. Participants or 'informants' are selected because they are people who are in the best position to understand the issues. Professional insights can be incorporated by including relevant interviewees and summary health data from primary and secondary care, but the principle of promotion of equality is at the heart of such an approach (Murray, 1999).

Table 3.4 Case studies

Case study 1	*Case study 2*
Community perceptions of health needs in south-east Edinburgh	*Mental health, alcohol and drugs health needs assessment using rapid participatory appraisal*
Objectives	**Objectives**
To assess public perceptions about local health needs and healthcare services and to gain views on how services could be improved	To assess the needs of individuals, their carers and the wider community with respect to mental health problems and to seek suggestions for service developments for service users and the wider community
Needs assessment team	**Needs assessment team**
An external researcher with community development training was assisted by a general practitioner. They intended to carry out a rapid appraisal but this was considered impractical as the area under study was large and comprised several communities, each of which could have been studied individually with rapid appraisal. Focus groups were used as an alternative, and these explored issues around the quality and coverage of primary care services	Comprised of a community psychiatric nurse (CPN), a general practitioner and psychiatrist. Interviews were carried out by the CPN
Time spent	**Time spent**
The outside researcher spent 2 days a week for 3 months on the study	The CPN spent 1 day per week for 4 months on the study

Setting

The area of study was in south-east Edinburgh (120,000 residents)

Results

Rapid appraisal could not be used as the area was too large but, more importantly, too diverse

Outcome

An alternative method was used, consisting of focus groups alone

Conclusions

Rapid appraisal could not be carried out without subdividing the area into natural communities where key informants are more likely to be knowledgeable about local problems. There were insufficient resources for this. Rapid appraisal works best in small homogeneous communities. Large communities are likely to be diverse

Setting

The rapid appraisal was carried out in a housing estate of 670 homes in central Edinburgh

Results

Rapid appraisal identified that many patients viewed their pressing problems as housing, employment and personal relationships rather than being related to health services. Residents and local workers were concerned at the high concentration of people with mental health, alcohol and drug-related problems in the area. A change in housing policy was considered the most useful intervention by many residents. A 'one-door' approach to health and social service provision was suggested

Outcome

A dialogue was initiated between the housing department and the local psychiatric directorate about clusters of mental illness within the locality to prevent mentally ill people from being 'ghettoised' and a drop-in club for the socially isolated was started in a community room

Conclusions

Rapid appraisal encouraged a holistic multidisciplinary approach to assessing the problems that mental illness, alcohol and drug use can create for individuals, their relatives and carers and the wider community.

A practice-based CPN may have an important role in the assessment of local needs. Rapid appraisal can be modified to focus on broad issues relating to specific groups of clients

---

ACTIVITY 3.4

Looking at the two case studies described together with what you have read about the use of rapid participatory appraisal, what potential advantages and limitations does a rapid participatory appraisal seem to offer when doing an HNA?

What underlying values can you identify?

Now consider two potential HNAs that could be undertaken in your local area. Using the headings in the case study, consider whether undertaking a rapid participatory appraisal would work for either of these two potential HNAs in your area. What results might you expect, and what outcome would be satisfactory? How might this approach complement other methods of HNA for the topics you have chosen?

If you can't identify any topics which are current in your area then think about the following:

- HNA of children and young people with language and communication problems;

- Housing needs of a neighbourhood with high levels of deprivation.

Comment

Rapid participatory appraisal is a community-oriented process which can lead to the development of links that continue beyond the appraisal process that may in turn facilitate change. Rapid appraisal techniques are based on principles of equity, participation and multiagency collaboration and acknowledge the need for local knowledge. Using a qualitative approach to gain an insight into a community's perspective of their own need in a short space of time (Bowling, 2000) and facilitating greater influence on the decisions about needs and how they should be prioritised are central to this approach. This involves drawing on a wide range of skills and resources both to carry out and to inform the assessment process (Sykes, 2009).

Two main disadvantages that are often associated with rapid participatory appraisals are the limited resources that are available and the timescale, which is often rather short. Murray (1999, p444) identifies a number of other limitations, such as the logistics of coordinating the project team involved and the need to ensure that potential bias is minimised. Murray (1999, p444) concludes that rapid appraisal is *best applied to a population that can be considered as a community in some sense of the word* and can be seen as providing *key pieces of the jigsaw but not the complete picture*.

Problem tree analysis

Problem tree analysis has been used effectively to identify key problems facing a community and is a well-developed tool used by many development agencies. It can be used to identify possible solutions to the key problems identified by mapping out causes and effects in a structured way. Key stakeholders are brought together to assess the current situation jointly. They are asked to identify the main problems facing their community and to suggest the causal relationships between these problems in a diagrammatic form – a problem tree (Figure 3.8).

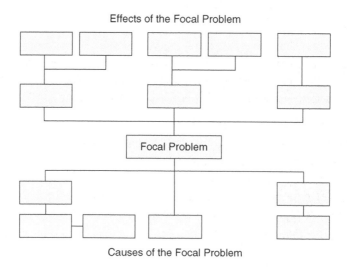

Figure 3.8 Structure of the problem tree, showing causes and effects

The process can be used to identify a range of problems identified by stakeholders or can be narrowed to focus attention on a specific problem area. For example, using this approach to identify the key health concerns, stakeholders would initially be asked to identify as many health problems as possible to get a complete overview of the situation. The next step is to reach consensus on what the stakeholders consider to be the main focal problem and then to proceed to identify direct causes of this problem. The next step involves identifying potential solutions to address the identified causes.

It would be easy to proceed through each of these steps and reach an early conclusion; however, all protagonists of the problem tree approach suggest that the heart of the exercise is the discussion and the generation of debate and dialogue about the problems, their causes and consequences and the subsequent generation of potential solutions.

Case Study: Problem tree analysis in practice

The following case study is an example of a problem tree that was developed through a series of workshops in a deprived community in the north-east of England (Figure 3.9).

The key focal problems identified by the stakeholders were high levels of long-term illness (mainly respiratory, heart disease and

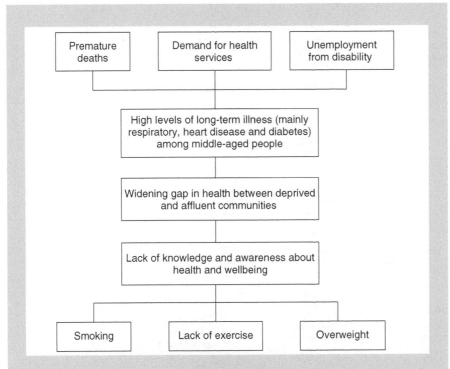

Figure 3.9 A problem tree developed in the north-east of England

diabetes) among middle-aged people, a widening gap in health status between deprived and affluent communities and a lack of knowledge and awareness of health and wellbeing.

In this example smoking, lack of exercise and increased numbers of people who are overweight were identified as direct causes of the problem, and premature death, increased demand for health services and increased unemployment as a result of disability as key effects or consequences of the problem. The next step involves identifying potential solutions to address the problems identified. This involves transforming the elements of the problem tree into an objectives tree by rephrasing each of the problems into desirable positive objectives and then reviewing these to look for realistic means to address them. The drawing enables visualisation of means–end relationships. Some objectives may seem unrealistic or too ambitious, whilst others will appear feasible within the context of the possible interventions (Overseas Development Institute, 2009).

Figure 3.10 is an example of an objectives tree based on a series of workshops in a deprived community in the north-east of England.

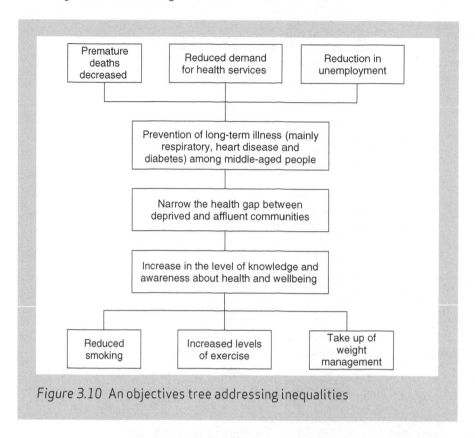

Figure 3.10 An objectives tree addressing inequalities

Chapter summary

In this chapter we began by considering what is meant by 'health', 'health needs' and 'health needs assessment'. Different types of HNA, such as comparative, corporate and epidemiological, were introduced and the relationship between HNA and the planning cycle explored. Two commonly used approaches to conducting an HNA – the two-stage approach and the five-step approach – were described. Rapid participatory appraisal and problem tree analysis were introduced as tools for increasing community involvement in HNA.

GOING FURTHER

Cavanagh, S and Chadwick, K (2005) *Health Needs Assessment.* London: Health Development Agency. Available online at: **www.nice.org.uk/media/150/35/Health_Needs_Assessment_A_Practical_Guide.pdf** (accessed 20 August 2012). *This updated guide to undertaking an HNA draws heavily from Hooper and Longworth's workbook (below). It is slightly less complex and updated to suit the external context better. A useful resource that provides practical guidance on doing an HNA.*

Hooper, J and Longworth, P (2002) *Health Needs Assessment Workbook*. London: Health Development Agency. Available online at: **www.nice.org.uk/niceMedia/ documents/hna.pdf** (accessed 20 August 2012).
This is a definitive guide to doing a basic need assessment and has stood the test of time. The authors identify five steps that need to be worked through when undertaking an HNA and provide clear guidance on how to work through each of these steps.

Stevens, A and Raftery, J (1994) *Introduction; Health Care Needs Assessment: The Epidemiologically Based Needs Assessment Reviews* (vol 1). Oxford: Radcliffe Medical Press. Available online at: **http://www.birmingham.ac.uk/ research/activity/mds/projects/HaPS/PHEB/HCNA/index.aspx**.
At this website you can find a link to the series and the 38 needs assessments that cover a range of diseases and populations in the references. This remains the best series on needs assessment by service (e.g. community child health) and topic (e.g. renal disease).

chapter 4

Health Surveillance

Rhonda Ware and John Harvey

Meeting the Public Health Competences

This chapter will help you to evidence the following competences for public health (Public Health Skills and Career Framework):

- Level 5(c): Knowledge of basic quantitative and qualitative methods of surveillance and assessment of the population's health and wellbeing;
- Level 5(e): Knowledge of the use of trend data in monitoring health and wellbeing and needs;
- Level 5(1): Collect and collate routine data on health and wellbeing and needs using a range of tools and techniques;
- Level 6(a): Understanding of how health and wellbeing, needs and outcomes are monitored;
- Level 6(3): Assess the implications of surveillance and assessment data relating to a defined population and recommend appropriate response(s);
- Level 7(6): Interpret and apply indicators for monitoring the population's health and wellbeing.

This chapter will also assist you in demonstrating the following National Occupational Standard for public health:

- Interpret data and information about health and wellbeing and/or stressors to health and wellbeing (PHP05).

This chapter will also be useful in demonstrating Standard 6 of the Public Health Practitioner Standards.

Standard 6

Obtain, verify, analyse and interpret data and/or information to improve the health and wellbeing outcomes of a population/community/group – demonstrating:

- b. knowledge of the main terms and concepts used in epidemiology and the routinely used methods for analysing quantitative and qualitative data;
- c. ability to make valid interpretations of the data and/or information and communicate these clearly to a variety of audiences.

Overview

This chapter will help you to understand the concept of health surveillance, and what is required to establish an effective system for carrying out relevant surveillance. You will understand the disease model on which health surveillance is based and the purposes for which it is used.

Exercises in this chapter will focus on:

- understanding and using a framework (causal pathway of disease or disability) to investigate and monitor a perceived problem;
- understanding and considering what data are needed to monitor and undertake health surveillance;
- designing a health surveillance survey and choosing appropriate measures;
- understanding and considering how to monitor incidence using a specific case study.

This chapter uses theory, tools and case studies to appreciate some of the key indicators and measures that are used in the surveillance and assessment of the population's health and wellbeing.

After reading this chapter you will be able to:

- define the purpose and components of health surveillance;
- understand what can be learnt from health surveillance;
- identify the main sources of information from surveillance programmes;
- assess the implications of surveillance data relating to a defined population or a defined setting, recommend appropriate public health actions and monitor their impact.

Health surveillance

Surveillance is one of the key public health roles, and involves following rates of disease and illness within a population and taking action to address unexpected variations. The purpose of surveillance is to guide and monitor public health policy and strategies. This includes informing the assessment of the status of health in a population, defining public health priorities, identifying topics for research and evaluation of public health programmes. The World Health Organization (WHO) has defined public health surveillance as *an ongoing, systematic collection, analysis and interpretation of health-related data essential to the planning, implementation, and evaluation of public health practice closely integrated with the timely dissemination of these data to those responsible for prevention and control* (CDC, 2010).

The objective of health surveillance activities is to take action that will help to control the health risk or condition under surveillance. A key principle is that appropriate action requires appropriate information. Surveillance systems therefore need to: be capable of functioning as an early-warning system; be able to identify public health emergencies and record the impact of an intervention or progress towards specified public health targets and goals; and support the understanding and monitoring of the epidemiology of a specified condition.

An effective surveillance system has the following components (WHO, 2010):

- detection and notification of health events;

- collection and consolidation of pertinent data;

- investigation and confirmation (epidemiological, clinical and/or laboratory) of cases or outbreaks;

- routine analysis and creation of reports;

- feedback of information to those providing the data;

- feed-forward (i.e. the forwarding of data to more central levels);

- feed-up (i.e. reporting data to the appropriate administrative level).

Detection and notification of health events

The key point here is the definition of the event, which may be a 'case' in clinical terms. The definition needs to be clear and the parameters should ensure that the 'event' is rightly identified and reported to the right place at the right time. The following case study provides an example to illustrate how this is applied in practice.

Case Study: Setting a case definition

Under the *International Health Regulations 2005* (WHO, 2008b), the WHO established case definitions for the following four critical diseases which are always deemed to be unusual or unexpected and may have serious public health impact, and hence must be notified to the WHO in all circumstances:

1. smallpox;
2. poliomyelitis due to wild-type poliovirus;
3. human influenza caused by a new subtype;
4. severe acute respiratory syndrome (SARS).

Case definition for notification of SARS under the IHR (2005)

In the SARS post-outbreak period, a notifiable case of SARS is defined as an individual with laboratory confirmation of infection with SARS coronavirus (SARS-CoV) who either fulfils the clinical case definition of SARS or has worked in a laboratory with live SARS-CoV or storing clinical specimens infected with SARS-CoV.

Clinical case definition of SARS

1. A history of fever, or documented fever

and

2. One or more symptoms of lower respiratory tract illness (cough, difficulty breathing, shortness of breath)

and

3. Radiographic evidence of lung infiltrates consistent with pneumonia or acute respiratory distress syndrome (ARDS) or autopsy findings consistent with the pathology of pneumonia or ARDS without an identifiable cause

and

4. No alternative diagnosis can fully explain the illness.

Source: www.who.int/ihr/Case_Definitions.pdf

Collection and consolidation of pertinent data

Good data management is critical to the success of health surveillance. Data management is a routine process that consists of a number of basic functions, including systematic collection and orderly consolidation of the data. The quality of the data is also important and there are some key criteria that need to be fulfilled. First, the data should be complete. From a data management perspective the data are complete if all reported cases of the disease and all the required details of each case are available. For example, take childhood immunisation: if all the child health clinics but only 75 per cent of general practitioner (GP) surgeries in a primary care trust send their vaccination and immunisation returns for entry on the child health information system (CHIS), the reported coverage will be low due to incomplete data. This could result in taking inappropriate action, such as trying to identify why the level of uptake (by parents) is low rather than considering why the surgeries have not returned their data.

Second, data should be accurate and reflect reported details correctly. Errors generally occur at three points: the primary record (usually clinical) may be wrong or unclear; the transcription to the notification form may include an error; or the data input to an electronic database may involve an error. Common sources of error are secondary coding (i.e. someone is interpreting the primary record to answer a question), incorrect dates, and incorrect patient identification, often leading to duplication.

Third, the data provided should be timely in order to enable effective action to be taken. The meaning of 'timely' depends on the objective of the surveillance activity. The timing requirements may be immediate, recent (up to 1 year), or longer term when future trends are monitored. An example of immediate need is when the surveillance activity is aimed at knowing whether there is increasing incidence of a condition such as influenza during the winter months. The data need to be timed to allow an estimate of the numbers week by week.

Monitoring of recent data may look at quarterly or annual figures, which should be available within weeks of the end of the period. An example is maternity data looking at perinatal morbidity and mortality. Longer-term data requirements are related to rarer events, such as a specific disease like Creutzfeldt–Jakob disease, where trends over years are monitored. Of course these categories are not mutually exclusive.

Other criteria for quality data include: appropriateness – the data need to be related to the surveillance activity; availability, which is self-explanatory; and the conciseness and presentation of the data – it needs to be in a form that is easily found and is clearly presented.

Investigation and confirmation (epidemiological, clinical and/or laboratory) of cases or outbreaks

Investigation and confirmation of cases or outbreaks is an important element of health surveillance. It may be carried out by the agency to which the event is reported, or may rely on the outcome of investigation at the source. Broadly there are three options:

1. If the case definition requires a clinical assessment (such as a GP diagnosing a flu-like illness) or a laboratory confirmation (such as human immunodeficiency virus (HIV) status), or certification of cause of death, the assumption is that reported cases are true cases.

2. If the cases are reported as a cluster, such as cases with symptoms indicating an outbreak of food poisoning, then epidemiological investigation and laboratory identification of any causative organism are required.

3. If the number of cases in a population exceeds the expected numbers, then an audit process is used to review and confirm the relevant clinical and epidemiological data. For example, investigating an upward trend in infant deaths in a population would require that the circumstances of death be considered.

Routine analysis and creation of reports

Regular production of reports is part of the surveillance activity. These should be produced in accordance with a standard format. The reports should be sent out promptly to the relevant people.

Feedback of information to those providing the data

This function is critical to sustaining the flow of complete and accurate information. This should involve both the data managers and the clinicians and allow discussion of the validity of the data as well as the implications in public health terms.

Feed-forward (the forwarding of data to more central levels)

The primary collection and consolidation of data may be carried out at local, regional or national levels. However the data may be collated at a larger population level, and require forwarding. For example, childhood immunisation coverage is collected at local level in the UK and forwarded to the regional office and nationally to the Department of Health; cancer registration is collated at a regional level and forwarded to the Office for National Statistics (ONS); data on pandemic flu cases is collated nationally and forwarded to the WHO.

Feed-up (reporting data to the appropriate administrative level)

Reports with the latest results should go to the persons who make or influence decisions, as well as to all who participate in the surveillance process and to other interested parties or organisations. For example, reports on perinatal and infant mortality should go to the Director of Public Health for the local area, who has responsibility to work with the commissioner(s) and provider(s) to address the key findings.

What should health surveillance include?

Health surveillance will focus on a number of different aspects of health and wellbeing, and the threats to health in particular. One useful way to consider the range of issues which should be subject to surveillance is to take as a model a causal pathway of disease or disability, as illustrated in Figure 4.1.

This model helps in the event of public or political pressure to investigate or monitor a perceived problem. If there is a plausible pathway that can be described and investigated, then health surveillance data may be a good source of information which can be analysed to address the issues.

The relationship between health surveillance and health needs assessment

Health surveillance systems contribute to health needs assessment in a number of different ways. In Chapter 1 there was an emphasis on the importance of robust public health models to frame health needs assessment. Key points included the determinants of health and wellbeing, especially the social determinants, the incidence and/or prevalence of disease, disorders or events given exposure to adverse

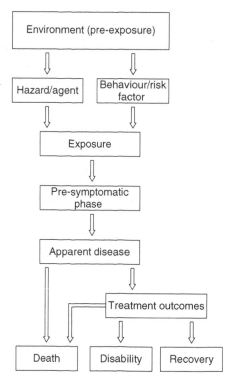

Figure 4.1 Model: causal pathway of disease or disability

Source: Adapted from CDC (2010).

ACTIVITY 4.1

Approximately 250,000 US children aged 1–5 years have blood lead levels greater than 10 micrograms of lead per decilitre of blood, the level at which the Centers for Disease Control and Prevention (CDC) recommend public health actions be initiated. (This level has recently been reduced to 5 μg/dl.) Lead poisoning can affect nearly every system in the body. Because lead poisoning often occurs with no obvious symptoms, it frequently goes unrecognised. Children are exposed in older houses in less affluent areas to lead from previous lead-based paints.

You have to set up a health surveillance system to monitor the efforts to reduce the exposure to lead. Using the model in Figure 4.1, decide what the pathway might involve and find out what elements of the causal pathway are subject to routine surveillance.

Outline the regular report you will send to local health departments.

Hint: look at the CDC's Childhood Lead Poisoning Prevention Program at **www.cdc. gov/nceh/lead/about/program.htm**

> **Comment**
>
> The causal pathway will involve the presence of lead (in paint or as a contaminant in dust and soil) and exposure to that through ingestion. As with any environmental hazard, you will want to measure the risk of exposure, incidence of presymptomatic conditions and incidence of symptomatic conditions with the outcomes of treatment. The sources on exposure will be local, state and federal (in the USA) household surveys, disclosures required on the sale of a property and incidents of non-compliance with disposal of lead-contaminated material. Medical laboratories will have data on raised blood levels of lead in your target population (children 5 years or younger) and healthcare providers or insurers will have a record of frank lead poisoning, for example, hospital admissions for treatment to lower blood lead levels. Your regular report will address these parameters and would highlight the effectiveness and urgency of primary prevention.

circumstances and the longitudinal impacts of adverse circumstances throughout the life course. Chapter 2 looked at measures and indicators that are critical for the monitoring and evaluation of the actions taken as a result of a health needs assessment. Table 4.1 illustrates some of the contributions health surveillance systems make to needs assessment.

Table 4.1 Health surveillance and health needs assessment (HNA)

HNA category	Available data	Source: surveillance agency
Determinants	Employment	National government – unemployment benefit
	Housing standards	Local authority housing survey
Incidence or	Prevalence of smoking	Health survey
prevalence	Incidence of lung cancer	Cancer registry
Longitudinal	Childhood obesity	National Child Measurement Programme
(analysis by risk group)	Suicide	Office for National Statistics

What can we learn from health surveillance?

The functions listed at the beginning of this chapter serve as a useful framework to check what surveillance might tell us. Here are some examples.

Serve as an early-warning system

The notification system for infectious diseases will identify a new disease (e.g. a new strain of flu) or an outbreak of a disease which is controlled, say by immunisation, such as measles.

Identify public health emergencies

At a global health level, the emergence of a pandemic situation due to a new virus will be shown up by the early-warning system. At a national and local level the shared information about cases of notified disease will alert the Health Protection Agency about a problem such as legionella infection, with a probable common source.

Record impact of an intervention or progress towards specified public health targets/goals

The impact of cancer screening programmes is assessed by the incidence (registration) of the specific cancer.

The targeting of an immunisation programme such as BCG (for tuberculosis) or hepatitis B will depend on the pattern of incidence in the population.

Understand/monitor the epidemiology of a specified condition (this may be achieved by a focused research study)

The registration of congenital anomalies allows studies of associations (e.g. with landfill sites) and factors such as maternal age.

Case Study: Congenital anomalies

EUROCAT is a European network of population-based registries for the epidemiologic surveillance of congenital anomalies (**www.eurocat-network.eu**). It was started in 1979, and there are 43 registries in 20 countries. More than 1.5 million births are surveyed per year in Europe (0.29 per cent of the European birth population). The registries are high-quality, multiple-source registries, ascertaining terminations of pregnancy as well as births.

The objectives of EUROCAT are:

- to provide essential epidemiologic information on congenital anomalies in Europe;
- to facilitate the early warning of new exposures to teratogenic agents (substances which are capable of interfering with the development of a fetus, causing birth defects);
- to act as an information and resource centre for the population, health professionals and managers regarding clusters or exposures or risk factors of concern.

This database allows researchers to look at specific trends. For example, gastroschisis is an abdominal wall defect more prevalent in the offspring of young mothers. It is known to be increasing in prevalence despite the general decrease in the proportion of births to young European women.

Using this database, Loane *et al.* (2007) investigated whether the increase in prevalence was restricted to the high-risk younger mothers. They analysed 936 cases of gastroschisis from 25 population-based registries in 15 European countries from 1980 to 2002.

The maternal age-standardised prevalence (standardised to the year 2000 European maternal age structure) increased almost fourfold from 0.54 per 10,000 births in 1980–84 to 2.12 per 10,000 births in 2000–02. The relative risk of gastroschisis for mothers <20 years of age in 1995–2002 was 7.0. There were geographical differences within Europe, with higher rates of gastroschisis in the UK, and lower rates in Italy after adjusting for maternal age. After standardising for regional variation, the results showed that the increase in risk over time was the same for mothers of all ages. These findings indicate that the phenomenon of increasing gastroschisis prevalence is not restricted to younger mothers.

(Adapted from Loane *et al.*, 2007)

Sources of data for health surveillance

The principles above have been put into practice in a variety of ways. Public health surveillance draws on a wide range of relevant data sources, involving a number of different methods of data collection.

There are three key methods of surveillance activity – through notification and registration processes, undertaking surveys and sentinel surveillance.

Notification/registration

This is a process whereby an informant is required to notify or register an event. In the case of a birth, for example, the informant for the purposes of civil registration is the parent. Registration of birth is mandatory by law. In cancer registration the informant is a health professional, often, but not necessarily, a clinician. Notification is a requirement to send information on an event to the appropriate authority or agency. For example, infectious disease notification is required by law in the UK and is made to the 'proper officer' of the local authority (either through the environmental health department or directly to the Health Protection Agency, which provides the proper officer function). In this instance the person responsible for notification is the registered medical practitioner who is involved in the diagnosis of the infectious disease. The local authority has to pass on that information to the Health Protection

'VERPOOL JOHN MOORES UNIVERSITY
LEARNING SERVICES

Agency within 3 days. Compliance with notification requirements varies considerably so the data may be incomplete.

Survey

Surveys were discussed in Chapter 2 as a method of gathering information about a population through observations, questionnaires, and so on. A good example of this is the Health Survey for England (HSE), which comprises a series of annual surveys that begun in 1991. This survey is now commissioned and published by the NHS Information Centre and is designed to provide regular information on various aspects of the nation's health. All HSE surveys have covered the adult population aged 16 and over living in private households in England. Children were included in every year since 1995. Each year the HSE focuses on a different demographic group and looks at health indicators such as cardiovascular disease, physical activity, eating habits, oral health, accidents and asthma. Surveys focusing on the health status of the population are carried out in other countries. The Welsh Health Survey and the Scottish Health Survey are similar to the England survey. In Northern Ireland there is a Continuous Household Survey.

The European Health Surveys Information Database (EUHSID) project maintained and updated a database of the characteristics of major Health Interview Surveys and Health Examination Surveys in Europe (accessed at: **www.euhsid.org**).

Sentinel surveillance

Sentinel surveillance provides an alternative to population-based surveillance for the collection and analysis of individual patient-related information and more limited monitoring of trends. The monitoring of predetermined health events is provided through sentinel sites or providers. For example, GP practices may be recruited on a voluntary basis to report particular conditions (such as an infectious disease, or long-term condition) for a fixed period. These data can be extrapolated to give indicative rates for incidence or prevalence.

Other monitoring systems and records are useful in the surveillance of health. These include environmental monitoring systems, individual health records, information on animal vectors, databases provided by laboratories, other administrative records and a whole range of records of adverse events. The information may be collected and collated through the above methods, or interrogated at source.

Environmental monitoring systems

These include air pollution monitoring carried out by local authorities, and water supply monitoring carried out by the local water company. Both sets of data are available through the Department for Environment, Food and Rural Affairs (Defra).

Animal vectors

Animals that are vectors for human disease and therefore present a risk to human health may be subject to surveillance. Obvious examples are mammals that may be carrying rabies, and insects capable of transmitting specific diseases, such as Lyme disease (which is tick-borne).

Individual health records

Individual health records are the source of identification of cases (by case definition) and may be found in paper or electronic records held in primary care (the GP clinical record system), hospitals (the patient administration or information system) or by other care providers.

Laboratories

Laboratories hold data on test results ranging from biochemical (such as blood lead levels), microbiological (such as identifying a strain of pneumococcus bacteria) to histological (such as a specific type of cancer) results.

Administrative records

Records collected for administrative reasons may have relevance to health and well-being. For example, records of people collecting unemployment benefits or on eligibility to free school meals provide relevant economic information.

Police records

The police collect data on several topics which are of interest in public health surveillance. For example, data on road traffic accidents, alcohol-related incidents and domestic violence are routinely used to inform public health policy.

Adverse events

Some industries may be required to report certain adverse events to the agency with particular (usually legally defined) responsibilities. For example, the Reporting of Injuries, Diseases and Dangerous Occurrences Regulations 1995 (RIDDOR) places a legal duty on employers, self-employed people and people in control of premises to report work-related deaths, major injuries or over-7-day injuries (not counting the day of injury), work-related diseases and dangerous occurrences (near-miss accidents) to the Health and Safety Executive within 15 days after the injury occurred. A pharmacist, doctor or patient can report a suspected adverse drug reaction or a side effect from a medicine or vaccine using the Yellow Card system to the Medicines and Healthcare products Regulatory Agency.

The principal agencies involved in health surveillance

There are a number of agencies which are central to health surveillance activity and without which the achievement of effective health surveillance would be compromised. The Association of Public Health Observatories (APHO) represents a network of 12 public health observatories (PHOs) working across the five nations of England, Scotland, Wales, Northern Ireland and the Republic of Ireland. The PHOs produce information, data and intelligence on people's health and healthcare for practitioners, policy makers and the wider community. Their expertise lies in turning information and data into meaningful health intelligence. The APHO and the PHOs all have policy lead areas, such as children, or mental health.

Cancer registries collect information about new cases of cancer and produce statistics about cancer-related incidence, prevalence, survival and mortality. The UK is widely acknowledged as having one of the most comprehensive cancer registration systems in the world. There are currently 11 cancer registries in the UK, each covering populations of between approximately 1.65 and 13.8 million people. Cancer registration in England is conducted by eight regional registries, which also submit a standard dataset of information to the ONS, for the collation of national cancer incidence data. Northern Ireland, Scotland and Wales each have one national cancer registry.

In the USA the CDC is dedicated to protecting health and promoting quality of life through the prevention and control of disease, injury and disability. The CDC seeks to accomplish its mission by working with partners throughout the nation and the world to monitor health, detect and investigate health problems, conduct research to enhance prevention, and develop and advocate sound public health policies.

Across Europe EUROCAT is a network of population-based registers for the epidemiological surveillance of congenital anomalies, covering 1.5 million births in 20 countries of Europe and EUROCARE (the European Cancer Registry-based study on survival and care of patients) is a cancer epidemiology research project that has a focus on the survival of European cancer patients. The project is based on a collaboration established in 1989 between two academic institutions in Italy and a large number of population-based cancer registries, from 12 European countries, with incidence and survival data available.

The Health Protection Agency, based in the UK, is responsible for providing information and services to support a coordinated and consistent UK public health response to national-level emergencies. Since its inception the Agency has provided specialist national, regional and local health protection services, including advice to others who also have health protection responsibilities. It maintains surveillance both nationally and internationally of potential threats and works with international partners to reduce the impact of threats to public health. The Agency provides reports on statutory notifications of infectious diseases. In England in April 2013 these responsibilities and those of the public health observatories will pass to Public Health England.

The NHS Information Centre is a central, authoritative source of health and social care information for England. In this role it collects, analyses and presents national data and statistical information in health and social care. This includes population health analysis and surveys, health screening, clinical quality and prescribing.

The ONS is the executive office of the UK Statistics Authority, a non-ministerial department which reports directly to Parliament. The ONS is the UK government's single largest statistical producer and provides independent information aimed at improving the understanding of the UK's economy and society. Reliable and impartial statistics are seen as vital for planning the proper allocation of resources, policy making and decision making to ensure a fair society.

The WHO is the directing and coordinating authority for health within the United Nations system. It is responsible for providing leadership on global health matters. The WHO fulfils its objectives through its core functions, which include: setting norms and standards and promoting and monitoring their implementation; providing technical support, catalysing change and building sustainable institutional capacity; and monitoring the health situation and assessing health trends.

ACTIVITY 4.2

A small coastal island community claims to have a cluster of cases of cancer. The residents put this down to the presence of petrochemical facilities very close to the island.

What data do you need to answer the questions raised?

Research the options (sources) for obtaining relevant data to monitor this problem. This will require searching websites provided by the above agencies, and finding others with a relevant remit.

Will the data that are available be enough to answer the questions? If not, what else would you like to know (ideally)?

Comment

The theoretical causal pathway would involve exposure to hydrocarbons, and the possible health impact would be seen in other conditions besides some types of cancer. Exposure could be from pollution of the air or land and water.

You would need to check with the local authority what monitoring data they hold on air quality and where it is collected. The government department responsible for environmental safety (the Environment Agency in the UK) should have a record of any incidents, such as large spills which might have put residents at risk, although these should also be known to the local-authority environmental health office. Defra is another website to search.

GPs may be aware of increased unexplained respiratory or neurological conditions, and the numbers could be obtained from practices. (Beware of problems of case definition, discussed above.) Admission rates for specific diseases may be useful. Look at the National Cancer Intelligence Network and the ONS for cancer and mortality data. Is it available at a small-area level on the website?

Would you get better information for another jurisdiction, like the USA, or from international organisation websites?

The small numbers of events in this case will make it difficult to answer the question as to whether there is a true excess, and the causal chain of possible exposure will not be fully refutable without biomedical tests to ascertain actual exposure. It would be possible to request an analysis at small-area level from the cancer registry responsible for the region.

Health surveillance systems

There are a number of health surveillance systems that have been established to provide comprehensive monitoring and surveillance. Two such examples are workplace (occupational) health and child health information systems (CHIS).

Occupational health

In the workplace health surveillance is about systematically watching out for early signs of work-related ill health in employees exposed to certain health risks. It means putting in place certain procedures to achieve this. In this context the purposes of health surveillance are:

- protection of health of the individual employee;

- detection at an early stage of any adverse health effects;

- assisting in the evaluation of control measures;

- data may be used for detection of hazards and assessment of risk;

- other purposes: for example, immune status assessment.

Case Study: Noise-induced hearing loss

Noise-induced hearing loss is irreversible and is one of the commonest occupational diseases. It is caused by exposure to sound levels such that the hair cells of the cochlea (inner ear) are damaged. Repeated exposure leads to a permanent decrease in hearing sensitivity, and an irreversible hearing loss.

Globally, 16 per cent of the disabling hearing loss in adults is attributed to occupational noise. The effects of the exposure to occupational noise are larger for males than females.

Employers have a legal duty to reduce the risk of hearing damage to their employees and there are actions which must be taken if noise exceeds certain defined limits. In the UK, the current regulations are the Control of Noise at Work Regulations 2005 (NaWR). The first action level is set at 85dB averaged over an 8-hour day. At this level, employers must provide information and training to employees on the health implications associated with noise. They must also make hearing protection equipment available.

The second action level is set at 90dB. Above this level, an employer must do all that is reasonably practicable to reduce noise levels, using whatever control measures are available. Until effective controls can be implemented, use of hearing protection is mandatory.

To put this in perspective, a normal conversation can register between 50dB and 60dB and a motorised garden tool can register between 115dB and 120dB.

Barlow and Castilla-Sanchez (2012) reported a study which measured noise exposure levels across a number of small-to-medium size (capacity -300–500) music venues where live and recorded music is played on a daily basis. Their objectives were to investigate:

- the actual level of noise exposure of employees in the venues under investigation;
- the level of understanding of the noise regulations among staff and management;
- the degree to which employers and employees in these venues adhered to the regulations.

When NaWR was put in place the music industry was included in the provision. They were given a 2-year window to respond to the requirements of the legislation, and from April 2008 the music and entertainment industries became regulated under the control of NaWR 2005. The regulations require employers in all areas of the entertainment industry to adhere to the same action levels for controlling noise exposure that apply to other industries such as working on a building site.

Barlow and Castilla-Sanchez (2012) say high levels of sound have traditionally been an integral part of both the live music industry and the nightclub industry, as this is considered an integral part of the experience. Noise levels in live popular music and rock concerts have been shown to be around 105–110dBA (decibel, adjusted using 'A-weighting' for sound response in the human ear) over the duration of a concert.

Their results showed that 70 per cent of the staff in all venues exceeded the daily noise exposure limit value (ELV) in their working shift. Of the bar and catering staff, more than half exceeded the ELV. None of the bar/catering staff at any venue wore any form of hearing protection at any time during the events being monitored nor could recall ever having used hearing protection at work. Of the technical staff, all of those listed as sound engineers (84 per cent of the group) were exposed to sounds in excess of the ELV during their working shift and 61.5 per cent of staff reported having been taught about the effects and levels of noise exposure at work. But 55 per cent of staff did not think that hearing protection was available in the venue. In all, 70 per cent of staff reported never using hearing protection, with 15 per cent using it occasionally, and 15 per cent regularly.

ACTIVITY 4.3

Thinking of the music industry, and the issues raised by the case study, describe a system of occupational health surveillance you would set up to monitor the impact of noise on the staff in a particular venue. Use the five points outlining the purpose of an occupational health surveillance as a framework.

Comment

The first part would be to record a risk assessment, using sound level meters and noise dosemeters. This will establish the extent of exposure and determine which employees are entitled to auditory testing on a regular basis. This is to detect any adverse health effects at an early stage. Statutory health surveillance is required for the protection of the hearing of workers exposed to high levels of noise, as required by NaWR 2005. It is applicable to:

- all employees working in defined hearing protection zones or regularly exposed to an averaged exposure over 85dBA;
- those employees regularly exposed to between 80 and 85dBA identified as being sensitive to noise-induced hearing loss.

The protection of health of the individual employee is achieved in part by control measures and the surveillance system will assist in the evaluation of control measures, and in part by the use of personal hearing protection, and you will want to monitor compliance in this regard.

In addition you should describe the record keeping you will set up to ensure health records of the health surveillance are carried out; that people who undertake health surveillance techniques are competent; and how and when people will be referred for further examination when their hearing tests show a problem and the results of those further tests with any treatment.

Child health information systems

In the UK a programme of child health surveillance has been in place since the early twentieth century. The programme has been revised several times. A programme based on a review of the evidence was introduced with the first edition of *Health for All Children* (Hall, 1989), produced by the Joint Working Party on Child Health Surveillance, which provided the basis for shaping future child health surveillance. The current programme was defined in October 2009 when the Department of Health issued the Healthy Child Programme. The rationale behind this was to provide comprehensive advice on health and social care throughout a child's life. The Healthy Child Programme differs from the previous schedule of child health surveillance in several key ways. First, there is an increased focus on antenatal care and a major emphasis on support for *both* parents. Another key difference is the early identification of at-risk families. New vaccination programmes have been included, such as the human papillomavirus (HPV) vaccine programme for girls aged 12–13, and there is a focus on changed public health priorities, such as strong parenting and child well-being, and readiness to learn.

The programme is delivered by a team that includes midwifery staff, health visitors and the primary care team, with GPs having responsibility for some newborn and the majority of 6–8-week checks. The programme places emphasis on the needs of at-risk families in response to an identified range of adverse outcomes for children (Social Exclusion Task Force, 2007). It is estimated that around 2 per cent of families in Britain experience five or more of the disadvantages identified in the list below.

- Both parents are unemployed.

- The family lives in poor-quality or overcrowded housing.

- Neither parent has any educational qualifications.

- Either parent has mental health problems.

- At least one parent has a longstanding limiting illness, disability or infirmity.

- The family has a low income.

- The family cannot afford a number of food and clothing items.

Surveillance in this programme requires a series of recorded contacts with the child and family. The outcomes are used to trigger an intervention for the individual where needed and for the collation of population-based data. This is achieved through the local CHIS, which can be used to fulfil operational, clinical and strategic functions. At an operational level the CHIS can be used to generate appointments for immunisations or regular checks. At a clinical level the CHIS can be used to identify an individual child's development. For example, the child's language development progress can be found. The CHIS can also be used strategically, for example, to provide routine reports on the immunisation coverage rate.

ACTIVITY 4.4

The range of child health surveillance services provided by the local community partnership trust is aimed at promoting the optimal development of typically developing children aged from birth to 3 years.

- How would you monitor the incidence of developmental delay in your population?
- What data will you collect?
- Who will provide the data, and how will it be collated?
- What problems do you anticipate in data quality and how will you manage those risks?

Comment

This activity illustrates the opportunity to have available routinely a measure which will inform need assessment through a mix of clinical activity in different settings as part of child health surveillance. The first thing is to agree a case definition for developmental delay with the senior clinical staff. The point of diagnosis is the primary source of the data. The CHIS should hold a longitudinal record for every child in the area. The diagnosis may be made in a community facility (child development centre) or in a paediatric clinic at a hospital. The trick is to ensure it is recorded on CHIS, either in a dedicated field or with a code so that the numbers can be retrieved.

There could be a scale of severity, and the incidence could be expressed by age of diagnosis.

The data quality issues will start with the primary source – is there ambiguity about the clinical assessment and diagnosis? This will affect the validity of the overall data. The transactions involved in transferring information (say in paper form from clinic to the clerks responsible for data input to the CHIS) and updating the central dataset can result in inaccuracy and incompleteness. You would want to audit the data flow and test the accuracy of the data at all points.

Case Study: Chronic disease risk factor surveillance

The WHO STEPwise approach to surveillance of chronic disease risk factors (STEPS) is a simple, standardised method for collecting, analysing and disseminating data in WHO member countries (WHO, 2011).

By using the same standardised questions and protocols, all countries can use STEPS information not only for monitoring within-country trends, but also for making comparisons across countries. The approach encourages the collection of small amounts of useful information on a regular and continuing basis.

One example is the Adult Risk Factor Surveillance programme. The WHO STEPwise approach to chronic disease risk factor surveillance provides an entry point for low- and middle-income countries to get started on chronic disease surveillance activities. It is also designed to help countries build and strengthen their capacity to conduct surveillance.

The STEPS instrument covers three different levels of 'steps' of risk factor assessment. These steps are:

1. questionnaire;
2. physical measurements;
3. biochemical measurements.

The STEPS manual provides a complete overview and guidance to sites wishing to implement the WHO STEPwise approach to chronic disease risk factor surveillance. It includes both general information and specific instructional material that can be used for:

- planning and setting up STEPS;
- training;
- data collection;
- data entry;
- data analysis and reporting.

See www.who.int/chp/steps/en for the instrument.

Some topics are expanded. For example, physical activity includes a question on sedentary behaviour.

The following question is about sitting or reclining at work, at home, getting to and from places, or with friends, including time spent sitting at a desk, sitting with friends, travelling in a car, bus, train, reading, playing cards or watching television, but does not include time spent sleeping.

How much time do you usually spend sitting or reclining on a typical day?

This case study illustrates the way in which surveillance methodology can be applied to risk rather than events, and the usefulness of collecting small amounts of information regularly. A similar approach is being taken in the UK to inform the risk stratification of people with long-term conditions.

Chapter summary

The essential considerations in setting up a public health surveillance system have been described in this chapter. Collection of relevant and appropriate data in health surveillance is central to achieving an effective health surveillance system. In this chapter we considered what health surveillance should include and looked at the relationship between health surveillance and health needs assessment. Effective health surveillance makes an enormous contribution to measuring and improving different facets of health and wellbeing. The purposes of health surveillance are wide-ranging and include the assessment of public health status in different populations and settings, enabling public health priorities to be defined locally, nationally and internationally, and evaluating public health actions.

GOING FURTHER

CDC (2010) *Overview of Public Health Surveillance*. Atlanta, GA: Epidemiology Program Office, Centers for Disease Control and Prevention. Accessed at: **www.cdc.gov/osels/ph_surveillance/nndss/phs/files/overview.ppt**
This PowerPoint presentation sets out the purpose and uses of public health surveillance and illustrates the uses with a wide range of real data. It provides an excellent overview (hence the title of the presentation!) and a broad set of topics where the data have relevance to monitoring and informing public health actions.

Lee, LM, Teutsch, SM, Thacker, SB and St Louis, ME (2010) *Principles and Practice of Public Health Surveillance*, 3rd edn. New York: Oxford University Press. Available online at: **www2.cdc.gov/PHTN/catalog/pdf-file/LESSON5.pdf** (accessed August 2012).

This book, which is available to read online, is a definitive discussion of the concepts and practical considerations relating to public health surveillance. It is a useful resource as it contains a number of practical activities that should help you to define public health surveillance and its critical components, and list the major considerations in starting a surveillance system.

chapter 5

Measuring Health Outcomes
Claire Bradford

Meeting the Public Health Competences

This chapter will help you to evidence the following competences for public health (Public Health Skills and Career Framework):

- Level 5(5): Interpret data on health and wellbeing within own area of expertise or practice;
- Level 5(d): Understanding of the relevance and use of measures of socioeconomic deprivation in population health and wellbeing analysis;
- Level 6(c): Understanding of strengths, uses, interpretation and limitations of various types of data relating to health and wellbeing, needs and outcomes;
- Level 7(2): Measure, analyse, compare and interpret the health and wellbeing and needs of various populations, communities and groups;
- Level 7(6): Interpret and apply indicators for monitoring the population's health and wellbeing;
- Level 7(a): Understanding of qualitative and quantitative sources and methods for measuring, analysing and interpreting health and wellbeing, needs and outcomes;
- Level 7(c): Understanding of the full range of qualitative and quantitative data sources and methods for measuring, analysing and interpreting health and wellbeing, needs and outcomes.

This chapter will also assist you in demonstrating the following National Occupational Standard for public health:

- Interpret data and information about health and wellbeing and/or stressors to health and wellbeing (PHP05).

This chapter will also be useful in demonstrating Standard 6 of the Public Health Practitioner Standards.

Standard 6

Obtain, verify, analyse and interpret data and/or information to improve the health and wellbeing outcomes of a population/community/group – demonstrating:

a. knowledge of the importance of accurate and reliable data/information and the anomalies that might occur;

b. knowledge of the main terms and concepts used in epidemiology and the routinely used methods for analysing quantitative and qualitative data;

c. ability to make valid interpretations of the data and/or information and communicate these clearly to a variety of audiences.

Overview

Health outcomes measurement and assessment are important aspects of the assessment of quality of care in today's health services. This chapter outlines the fundamentals of outcome measurement, their strengths and weaknesses, and will help you to understand the importance of context in health outcomes measurement. Outcomes are not a new concept, though you could be forgiven for thinking the NHS had just discovered the idea, so the historical introduction sets the chapter in context.

After reading this chapter you will:

- understand the historical context of outcomes measurement;
- be able to define what is meant by health outcomes;
- understand the benefits and risks of outcomes measurement;
- have a framework for the assessment of abnormal outcomes.

Historical context

Health outcomes have a long history of importance. During the Crimean War (1853–56), Florence Nightingale established a clinical outcomes study for the deaths of soldiers. Upon arrival in the Crimea she was appalled at the disorganisation and standards of hygiene. She reorganised the system of care and improved cleanliness. The high mortality rates did not improve, however, until after sewers were cleared and ventilation improved. Using data collected on season and causes of death she was able to show that the likely cause of excess deaths was due to poor living conditions rather than her original hypothesis of poor nutrition. She was also able to show that soldiers in peace time had an excess of mortality. She was however not keen on mortality outcomes as indicators of quality of care:

> If the function of a hospital were to kill the sick, statistical comparisons of this nature would be admissible. As, however, its proper function is to restore the sick to health as speedily as possible, the elements which really give information as to whether this is done or not, are those which show the proportion of sick restored to health, and the average time which has been required for this object.
>
> (Nightingale, 1863, p4)

Another early adopter of the concept of the importance of health outcomes was Codman (1934), a Boston orthopaedic surgeon who developed the *end result idea*. He suggested:

The common sense notion that every hospital should follow every patient it treats, long enough to determine whether or not the treatment has been successful, and then to inquire 'if not, why not?' with a view of preventing similar failures in the future.

(Codman, 1934, ppV–XL)

This idea is recognisable as care pathway audit today. Codman's audit system was successful in demonstrating the outcomes of his patients but was unfortunately not taken up by his colleagues or the hospital in general.

Codman's contribution, however, was recognised by a more recent and well-known pioneer in the use of health outcomes – Donabedian (1989). In 1966 Donabedian described three distinct aspects of quality in healthcare: outcome, process and structure. He had misgivings about solely using outcomes as a measure of quality and cautioned that outcomes measurement cannot distinguish efficacy from effectiveness: that is, outcomes may be poor because the right treatment is badly applied or the wrong treatment is carried out well. *Outcomes, by and large, remain the ultimate validation of the effectiveness and quality of medical care* (Donabedian, 1966).

Donabedian also stated that outcomes measurement must always take into account the context. For example, factors other than the intervention may be very important in determining outcomes, and also the most important outcomes may be the least easy to measure, so easily measured but irrelevant outcomes are chosen (e.g. mortality instead of disability).

The NHS White Paper *Liberating the NHS* placed great emphasis on outcomes (Department of Health, 2010a). The consultation paper *Transparency in Outcomes: A Framework for the NHS*, published in England in 2010 (Department of Health, 2010c), outlined proposals for an outcomes framework made up of a focused set of national outcome goals that provide an indication of the overall performance of the NHS and are discussed later.

Defining health outcomes

There are many definitions of health outcomes but they all involve a change in health status. Some health outcomes relate to a specific population, group or community, whilst others specify that health outcome as a result of specific interventions. A clear example of this is provided by Frommer *et al.* (1992, p135), who define a health outcome as a *change in the health of an individual, group of people or population which is attributable to an intervention or series of interventions.*

Measurement of health outcomes requires the identification of the context, measurement of health status before an intervention undertaken, recording of intervention and measurement of health status again (i.e. three dimensions: context, intervention as well as health outcomes). It is important that any measured change in health status can be causally linked to the intervention applied. These stages address specific data requirements, as set out in Table 5.1.

Table 5.1 Four stages of data requirements for measuring outcomes

Identification of the context	What is the diagnosis? Description/demographics of the patient – age, gender, ethnicity
Measurement of the health status of the patient before intervention	Stage of the disease, other illnesses/comorbidities, level of disability
Recording of intervention	Medical, behavioural or surgical intervention given, supportive care required, routine treatment or clinical trial
Remeasurement of health status	Presence of disease or disability post-intervention, side-effects of intervention, death, patient-reported outcome

Health outcomes are measures that the users of health services have a right to access. Mortality data have become more and more openly available and are used as a proxy for health outcomes in hospitals. In 2005 a landmark publication set out mortality by named individual heart surgeons. The audit looked at low- and high-risk patients in an attempt to inform the public about the complexities of this type of analysis (Bridgewater, 2005). Dr Foster, the independent agency set up by Imperial College, London, publishes standardised mortality rates for hospitals regularly online with a view to empowering patients with relevant information.

However the reservations on the use of mortality data already expressed continue to apply today in the assessment of health services. In general, health outcomes measurement should be based on routine morbidity rather than mortality, not least because death is fortunately a relatively rare outcome given the high numbers of interventions applied daily in a modern health service.

Principles of routine health outcomes measurement

There are a number of principles that should underpin the collection of routine health outcomes measurement in order to produce consistent measures. These include the following.

- All three dimensions (context, intervention as well as outcomes) must be measured. It is not possible to understand outcomes data and give a reasonable interpretation without all three of these.

- Different perspectives on outcomes need to be acknowledged. For instance, patients, carers and clinical staff may have different views about which outcomes are important and desirable, and how you would measure them reliably.

- Prospective and repeated measurement of health status is superior to retrospective measurement of change, which relies on interpretation of data which may have been recorded for another purpose, and at worst, memory.

- The reliability and validity of any measure of health status must be known so that their impact on the assessment of health outcomes can be taken into account. *Reliability* is the consistency of a set of measurements or, in this case, indicators. *Validity* or accuracy is the degree to which a measurement truly measures the issue of interest.

- Data collected must be fed back to the *source* of the data to maximise data quality, reliability and validity. This is an important part of the audit cycle. Feedback should be of content (e.g. relationship of outcomes to context and interventions) and of process (data quality of all three dimensions).

Risks and benefits of routine health outcomes measurement

Routine health outcomes measurement carries a number of risks as well as benefits. The use of aggregated anonymised health outcomes data enables the collation of data on the effectiveness of interventions undertaken. This could be used to demonstrate the actual benefits in everyday clinical practice of interventions previously tested by randomised clinical trials. Health outcomes measurement can also be used to demonstrate benefit in situations where interventions either have not been or cannot be tested in randomised controlled trials such as the introduction of a new type of joint replacement prosthesis into routine clinical practice. Similarly, it is possible to identify relatively rare outcomes from previously unknown hazardous interventions that are only apparent in large datasets, such as the congenital abnormalities discussed in Chapter 4.

Another benefit is that it is possible to identify differences between clinical services with a similar case mix. This in turn can stimulate a search for testable hypotheses that might explain these differences and lead to improvements in treatment or management. The first assumption might be that standard or good practice is not followed in every case. The Quality Outcomes Framework in primary care is a clear example of this. The data show variation between practices and individual doctors on measures such as the number of people recorded with a (recent) blood pressure measurement, or the proportion of people with diabetes who have a biochemical marker, which is at or below the target value.

Other benefits of health outcomes measures include providing an opportunity to compare the outcomes of treatment and care from different perspectives such as patients and clinicians. Where patient-related outcome measures are used, data about individual patients can be used to track changes during treatment over periods of time. This can be particularly useful where treatment is taking place over a long period of time and where a number of different clinical teams are involved. Finally, such measures can be used to improve clinical practice when used as part of the audit cycle.

There are, however, a number of potential limitations and problems associated with the use of health outcome measures. For example, using outcomes data to commission services has considerable risk as the potential for introducing bias is high. Paying inadequate attention to the analysis of context data such as the case mix can lead to dubious conclusions. If data are not fed back to clinicians participating then data quality (and quantity) could fall below the thresholds necessary for reasonable interpretation. Where only a (small) proportion of episodes of healthcare have completed outcomes data, these data may not be representative of all episodes, although the threshold for this effect will vary from service to service, measure to measure. Being aware of these potential limitations is the first step to overcoming them. The case study below provides a practical example of using health outcomes to explore public concerns about the risk associated with a particular health service.

Case Study: Maternity services outcomes

A local newspaper raised concerns about the number of deaths of babies at a local maternity unit. This occurred in an area with an active surveillance and monitoring system for perinatal mortality. It was therefore possible to analyse the numbers and causes of death to determine if there was a cause for concern relating to care at the hospital.

Perinatal mortality rate definitions:

- stillbirth: *in utero* death delivering after the 24th week of gestation;
- early neonatal death: death of a live-born baby less than 7 completed days from time of birth;
- perinatal mortality rate: number of stillbirths and early neonatal deaths per 100 live births and stillbirth.

A control chart analysis for the hospitals in the area covered by the surveillance system showed that the maternity unit concerned had a perinatal mortality rate that was at the 3 standard deviation limit and therefore is classified as an alert which should be investigated (Figure 5.1). Statistical process control methodology based on control charts has been used for many years. It is designed to study variability over time or between institutions or areas and is a powerful tool for population health surveillance and monitoring (Flowers, 2007).

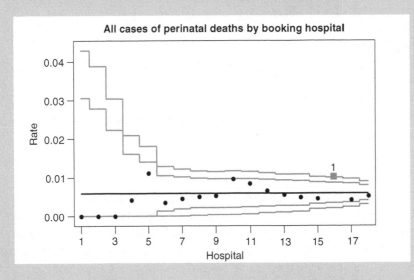

Figure 5.1 Control chart of perinatal mortality rates by maternity unit

Source: Regional Maternity Survey Office, North East Public Health Observatory.

95

The maternity unit instituted an investigation and analysis of deaths in the hospital over the relevant years. The investigation concentrated on deaths at full term and analysed 14 individual cases. Analysis of these cases included maternal age, body mass index at booking visit, gestational age at delivery and birth weight. There were ten ante-partum deaths, two intrapartum deaths and two early neonatal deaths. A cause of death was known for 12 cases, of which the majority ($n = 6$) was idiopathic antepartum hypoxia. In seven cases avoidable causes of a poor outcome were identified. Particular areas for improved care identified included education and training in relation to identification of intrauterine growth retardation and review of the local policy for induction of labour. A system of continued case review with critical incident analysis was implemented.

ACTIVITY 5.1

Think of the ways in which this study illustrates the principles of routine health outcomes measurement described earlier.

- What is the context?
- What are the interventions, and what is recorded about the health status of the mother and infant, before and after the intervention?
- What is the patients' (parents') perspective?
- What is the public view?
- Will clinical staff have different views about which outcomes are important?
- What information would you expect to be recorded prospectively?
- What will contribute to the reliability and validity of any measure of health status in this context?
- How will the data be fed back to the source of that data?

In considering your answers to these questions, what can you conclude here about using health outcomes?

Comment

The context is clear – in this example this is the 'events' which are counted in calculating perinatal mortality, and one of the important aspects of the analysis is demography of the mothers. These events are defined in the case study. These rates are used commonly as outcomes for maternity services, and infant mortality (which includes early neonatal deaths) is used as an international comparator.

The interventions include a range of activities provided as part of antenatal care, and the management of the birth (intrapartum care). The health status of the mother is usually recorded in relation to factors which are associated with risk, such as maternal age, obesity or smoking in pregnancy. After birth, other factors such as breastfeeding and mental health status may be recorded.

For the infant, the important aspect of health status recorded *in utero* is the estimate of growth against a normative standard. At birth the birth weight and Apgar score (a composite measure of vital parameters) are recorded along with the critical issue of number of weeks' gestation. Specific conditions such as congenital anomalies and respiratory disorders are recorded. These make it possible to analyse causes of perinatal mortality and identify avoidable risk factors.

The parents' perceptions will be determined by their experience directly or indirectly of losing a baby in the perinatal period. Risk is explained, especially in high-risk pregnancies, where extra visits to antenatal clinics or indeed hospitalisation are required. It is probable that prospective parents will look at the performance of local maternity units to decide where they want to book for delivery where they have more than one accessible hospital.

Public perception is less easy to predict.

Professional views in the maternity services will often be determined by the relative rate of the local unit compared with regional or national rates. Whereas this may give the impression of complacency, this is a common (and flawed) way of 'benchmarking' in the NHS (see Chapter 6). However the maternity unit is concerned primarily to understand where perinatal deaths can be avoided, and the lessons learnt from local reviews and national confidential enquiries will be implemented as part of continuous quality improvement.

The quality of data will be improved by sharing in a regional or national data collection process which uses a standard protocol and gives regular feedback to midwives and doctors. A good example is the work of the West Midlands Perinatal Institute (**www.perinatal.nhs.uk**).

Measuring hospital mortality

We mentioned above that hospital mortality is collated and published as a way of informing the public about the performance of a given hospital compared with others. A hospital death rate is the number of people who die in hospital relative to its 'population'. If we want to know if the death or mortality rate is higher or lower than average or how hospitals compare, it is common to use a standardised mortality ratio (SMR), which is calculated by dividing the total of observed deaths by the total of expected deaths (see Chapter 1). In this example the number of deaths in hospital within a given time period is divided by the number that might be expected if the hospital had the same death rates as some reference population, e.g. the hospitalised population of England. As well as adjusting for age, most hospital mortality measures attempt to make adjustments for differences in gender, diagnosis, deprivation, comorbidity, whether the patient is recorded as receiving palliative care and sometimes the procedures that the patient has had. All these factors can influence deaths in a hospital but are outside its control, and therefore may confound any findings from an analysis of specific rates.

Interpreting hospital mortality ratios

By adjusting for age, gender, diagnosis and other factors, any remaining difference between a hospital's expected number of deaths and the actual number of deaths may be attributed to things within the hospital's control, such as quality of care. However, given the complex nature of the calculations involved and the various methods used, there are some important issues for hospitals to consider when interpreting this type of mortality measure before deciding what actions to take. It is essential to understand the relevant local service issues. We look at two key issues here: place of death and data quality.

Place of death

All hospitals serve a population. Within that population there will be alternative locations where someone may die; for example, at home, or in a hospital, hospice or care home. The higher the proportion of deaths which occur in hospital compared with the national average, the higher the hospital mortality ratio will be. Analysis carried out by Public Health Observatories and the National End of Life Care Intelligence Network (NEoLCIN) shows that the proportion of deaths in different settings varies widely from place to place depending on both the local area as well as the diagnosis. It is suggested that these variations can explain some of the difference between different hospitals' mortality ratios (NEoLCIN, 2010).

What's the evidence?

The Association of Public Health Observatories published a report *Dying to Know: How to Interpret and Investigate Hospital Mortality Measures* (APHO, 2010b) that sets out guidance for the use of hospital mortality data.

The use of SMRs has become an increasingly common way to monitor the performance of hospitals and their quality of care. However these measures have been the source of controversy. The hospital mortality ratio is at best similar to the smoke alarm in your house – it may signal something serious or it may 'go off' for reasons unrelated to quality of care. However, like your smoke alarm, they should not be ignored.

Every year around half a million people die in England (475,000 deaths were recorded in 2008). The proportion of those who died in hospital in 2008 was 58 per cent. These numbers and proportions have fallen since 2001. These figures do not help us to understand if this is due to improved quality of care. We need to calculate and compare death rates in order to enable hospitals to:

- reduce mortality rates;
- improve patient safety;
- reduce avoidable variation in care and outcomes.

Data quality

The quality of the available data is affected by data recording and clinical coding practice. Variations in how the place of death is recorded, palliative care coding, the depth of coding and general accuracy and variation in clinical coding all contribute.

How place of death is recorded

Counting the number of deaths in a hospital is not as straightforward as it may seem and what is included in the mortality statistics can vary from hospital to hospital. Most hospital mortality measures are based on the Hospital Episode Statistics (HES) dataset. HES contain records for inpatients and therefore count people who are admitted and who then die. Hospitals themselves often include in their data deaths which have occurred outside the hospital, for example, road traffic accidents, cardiac arrests outside hospital and those who die in Accident and Emergency units. These deaths will not have been influenced by the quality of care provided by the hospital.

Palliative care coding

At present there is no standard method of including palliative care patients in calculations of standardised hospital mortality ratios. There is a standard code for palliative care but there is great variability in its use. This is a good example of needing to know the local context in order to interpret different outcomes. If a ratio is used which takes account of the coding of palliative care and both mortality and coding levels are high, then this suggests that the explanation for a high mortality rate does not relate to poor-quality hospital care.

Depth of coding

Some mortality ratios include comorbidity or case mix measures which give an idea of the complexity and severity of cases. These measures are used to capture differences which influence patients' survival, such as comorbidities. The calculation of these depends on the recording of secondary or additional diagnoses.

Data quality audits at hospitals have shown that there is variation in the degree to which hospitals code for secondary diagnoses. The average number of diagnosis per patient is known as the depth of coding; the greater the depth, the greater the potential reduction in mortality rate if case mix adjustment is used. However, if mortality and depth of coding are not high then this will not be the explanation. Similarly, hospitals with average or low mortality ratios but a good depth of coding may be better at recording relevant codes, but this may disguise a genuinely high mortality rate.

Accuracy and variation in clinical coding

Some mortality ratios do not include all deaths (sometimes only around 80 per cent of all in-hospital deaths), including instead only deaths of people who have been admitted for certain reasons. Hospitals may code the reasons for an admission differently. This may bias the results of hospital mortality calculations. There are other important issues, including the use of particular case mix scores which rely on the completeness and accuracy of secondary diagnosis codes in HES (see Chapter 2).

Knowing when to act

SMRs and mortality rates vary between hospitals and fluctuate over time with hospitals. This is especially true if SMRs or mortality rates are monitored frequently over short periods of time. The degree of fluctuation will be higher simply because the effect of chance is greater when the number of deaths is smaller.

One basic consideration is whether the SMR is actually high, or is it just 'noise'? For SMRs the baseline is usually set at 100 and that means hospitals can calculate limits within which it would expect local mortality rates to sit. These limits are called control limits and can be set to different levels but are generally set so that the chance of exceeding these limits is about 1 in 1,000. If the local SMR is higher than the upper limit it may be a cause for concern. However, if it is below the lower limit it might also warrant attention – perhaps to identify and understand good practice, or data issues, e.g. coding inconsistency.

Trends and triggers

It is important to recognise that a single figure in time cannot be looked at in isolation – it must be examined in the context of a trend. For example, if a hospital's SMR for a single period does not exceed the control limits (3 standard deviations from the group average), but is persistently above 100, there may still be cause for concern.

Any of the following three scenarios, where there is a high chance that the pattern of the data has not risen by chance alone, could be used as a trigger for investigating a high mortality rate:

1. higher than the upper control limit on a single occasion;

2. higher than 100 on six or more successive occasions;

3. six or more consecutive increases, regardless of the start level (a rising trend).

Case Study: Mid-Staffordshire hospital

The Francis Inquiry (Department of Health, 2010b) was an independent inquiry commissioned by the Secretary of State for Health to investigate care given at the Mid-Staffordshire NHS Foundation Trust. There had been a number of previous investigations which had been as a result of concerns related to increased mortality rates at the hospital. This case study outlines the mortality rates which gave rise to concerns.

The initial concerns were raised in 2007 about the trust's mortality rate as compared with other similar trusts. The Dr Foster Hospital Guide showed that the trust had a higher than expected hospital SMR (HSMR) for 2005–06. In October 2007 the trust was assessed as 'good to fair' in the Healthcare Commission's (HCC) 2006–07 annual health check.

In April 2008 the HCC launched an investigation into the trust following what it regarded as a concerning reaction by the trust to the mortality statistics. The HCC's investigation turned out to be protracted. In March 2009 it published the report of its investigation, which was highly critical of the acute care provided by the trust.

A summary of the mortality statistics used in the various investigations is given in the Francis report. It was taken from a House of Commons report and is reproduced on page 5 of the report.

In addition the inquiry report provides an extract of the trust's own mortality surveillance. This showed significantly higher than expected mortality rates in ten areas. The statistical likelihood of these all being due to chance or coding errors is extremely unlikely.

The inquiry report states that:

> It will have been seen that on virtually every measure the Trust's results were statistically significantly higher than expected. It had a higher number of alerts, and its HSMR and SMR results were significantly high. Even the crude mortality rates were high.
>
> (Francis, 2010, p36)

The analysis in the Francis report is an excellent example of how mortality statistics can be used to highlight concern about the delivery of clinical care. It also explains how these statistics can only be of assistance if they are used in an enquiring and open manner.

Health status outcome measures

In order to provide a baseline for monitoring the health and social wellbeing of a population, a standardised generic measure of health is needed that would facilitate the collection of a common dataset and allow comparisons between different

---

ACTIVITY 5.2

Find the quality accounts for your local NHS trust providing acute care, and those of the neighbouring areas. Look for references to hospital mortality rates, and ask whether the trust has addressed any of the questions below. (They provide a checklist for investigating a high SMR.)

- How were the mortality rates measured and mortality ratios constructed? Is there enough information, or are the results presented in such a way as to distinguish a warning 'signal' from 'noise'?
- How would you investigate coding practices and check the underlying data?
- What are the key aspects of local palliative and terminal care services provision, including how hospital/community/other services are configured, which pathways are in use?
- What regular quality improvement tools could the trust use? How does the trust review hospital performance on a regular basis?
- Does the quality account include perinatal mortality information? If so, what does it show? If not, ask why not?

Comment

The mortality rates/ratios used in the quality accounts should state the source, whether calculated locally or from a national source. In either case the methodology should be explained briefly (especially as this is a public document). A good-quality account will have a section on data quality, which will tell you about the way the organisation is dealing with the factors which will improve the quality of the information. The local arrangements for intermediate care and end-of-life care will determine to some extent how many deaths will take place at home or in the community, and how many occur in hospital.

The trust should have regular mortality reviews and case note reviews, and use trigger tools (use of triggers to point up adverse events). The quality improvement programme should look at the HSMR, crude mortality rates and diagnosis-specific rates as part of a package of general quality improvement measures. The programme of clinical audit (also reported in the quality account) should be related in part to the issues which the outcome data are highlighting.

Finally, despite providing maternity services, there is no requirement to include outcomes from maternity service in the account. A good trust would include those rates as they are of major importance.

---

populations or subgroups. Since the 1970s, a number of instruments have been designed to be used as general purpose measures of health, independent of diagnostic categorisation or disease severity. The most widely used is the Short Form questionnaire, known as SF-36, developed to measure health outcomes from a patient perspective. Other instruments, such as the EuroQol EQ-5D questionnaire, General Health Questionnaire (GHQ-12) and patient-reported outcome measures (PROMs) are also used to measure health outcomes.

These instruments focus on aspects that may influence 'quality of life', such as ability to perform everyday activities, patient satisfaction with levels of functioning and control of disease, gap between expectations and achievements, the functional effect of an illness and consequent therapy, overall satisfaction with life and general sense of wellbeing and position in life in relation to goals and expectations in context of cultural values. The instruments are tested for validity (the degree to which a scale measures what the user intends it to measure) and reliability (the extent to which the measure yields the same number or score each time it is administered). However, many of the measures used in these instruments are country-specific and their validity for use as cross-cultural tools has been called into question (Anderson *et al.*, 1993). An exception to this is the EuroQol EQ-5D questionnaire, which was developed by an international research network established in 1987. A summary of each of the key instruments used is provided in the next section.

Summary of instruments used to measure health status outcome

SF-36

The SF-36 is a multipurpose, short-form health survey with 36 questions. It yields an eight-scale profile of functional health and wellbeing scores as well as psychometrically based physical and mental health summary measures and a preference-based health utility index. It is a generic measure, as opposed to one that targets a specific age, disease or treatment group. It was developed to monitor medical care outcomes, and is focused on the patient's point of view. Some criticisms include the view that brevity could lead to loss of precision, and that it omits concepts such as family function and sexual function.

The eight domains cover physical functioning; social functioning; role limitation – physical problems; role limitations – emotional problems; mental health; energy/vitality; pain; and perceptions of general health.

Typical questions asked focus on the extent to which health status is perceived as limiting a range of everyday activities. Figure 5.2 illustrates some of the questions used.

EuroQol EQ-5D

EQ-5D is a standardised instrument for use as a measure of health outcome. The EuroQol website says: *it is applicable to a wide range of health conditions and treatments; it provides a simple descriptive profile and a single index value for health status* (**www. euroqol.org**).

From the outset, the EuroQol Group has been multicountry, multicentre and multidisciplinary. The focus of EuroQol has been global and one of its key aims was to create the capacity to generate cross-national comparisons. It was originally designed to be self-completed by the respondent, making it ideal for use in a postal survey.

a. Does your health limit you in these activities? If so, how much?
- Vigorous activities
- Climbing several flights of stairs
- Walking more than half a mile
- Bathing and dressing yourself

Answers: Yes, limited a lot/yes, limited a little/no, not limited at all

b. How much bodily pain have you had during the past 4 weeks?

Answers: None/very mild/mild/moderate/severe/very severe

c. During the past 4 weeks, have you had any of the following problems with your work or other regular activities as a result of any emotional problems (such as feeling anxious or depressed)?

Answers:
- Cut down on the **amount of time** you spent
- **Accomplished less** than you would like
- Didn't do work or other activities as **carefully** as usual.

Figure 5.2 Typical questions used in the SF-36 health survey instrument

The EuroQol EQ-5D is a two-part measure, where the first part is a descriptive system which defines current health state in terms of five dimensions: mobility; self-care; usual activities; pain/discomfort; and anxiety and depression. Each dimension has three levels of severity (no problem; moderate problems; extreme problems) and respondents select one level of severity for each dimension to describe their current health. Typically 40 per cent of respondents in the UK report moderate problems in at least one dimension, and 5 per cent report severe problems.

The second part of the EuroQol EQ-5D consists of a vertical 20 cm, 0–100 visual analogue scale (VAS) like a thermometer, where 0 represents the worst imaginable health state and 100 represents the best imaginable health state. Respondents are asked to mark a point on the scale to reflect their overall health on that day. Together, the two parts of the EuroQol EQ-5D provide descriptive information about each of the five Euro-Qol dimensions and quantitative information about respondents' rating of their own health. A comparison of mean VAS scores in five populations is shown in Figure 5.3.

The VAS discriminates between different population groups by social class classification and by age group, as shown in Figure 5.4.

GHQ-12

A series of 12 questions that relate to the mood and affect of the respondent are sometimes used as a single instrument. These questions comprise the short-form GHQ-12, which is commonly used as a screening tool to determine anxiety and depression (Goldberg, 1972). The response categories to the GHQ are coded 0-0-1-1, with possible scores ranging from 0 (the lowest probability of having problems of anxiety or depression) to 12 (the highest probability). A score of 4 or above was

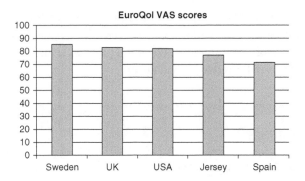

Figure 5.3 Mean EuroQol visual analogue scale (VAS) scores for different population groups

Sources: Sweden (Brooks *et al.*, 1991); United Kingdom (Kind *et al.*, 1998); United States (Johnson and Coons, 1998); Jersey (Gordon *et al.*, 2001); Catalan, Spain (Badia *et al.*, 1998).

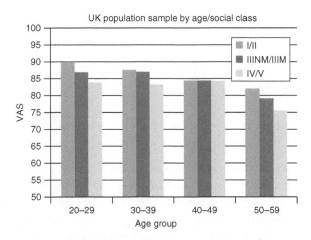

Figure 5.4 EQ-5D as a self-rated index (using EQ visual analogue scale (VAS) scores)

Source: Adapted from Kind *et al.* (1999).

suggestive of anxiety or depression. This simple tool maps well to the diagnostic classification of mental health disorders.

PROMs

PROMs measure quality from the patient perspective. Initially covering four clinical procedures, PROMs calculate the health gain after surgical treatment using pre- and postoperative surveys.

The four procedures chosen for the national pilot studies were hip replacements, knee replacements, hernia and varicose veins. Since April 2009, all providers of NHS-funded care have been required to collect PROMs for these four clinical areas. Patients are given pre- and postoperative questionnaires when they receive treatment for the four procedures above.

For each of these procedures the patient's health status or health-related quality of life is measured. This typically involves completion of short, self-completed questionnaires, which measure the health status or health-related quality of life at a single point in time. The health status information collected from patients by way of PROMs questionnaires before and after an intervention provides an indication of the outcomes or quality of care delivered to NHS patients.

What's the evidence?

Review of health status measures for PROMs

A structured review of PROMs for people with heart failure looked at ratings of the evidence of measurement and operational performance, applying the agreed appraisal criteria for PROMs to all of the available evidence. Based on this appraisal, the following instruments were recommended for consideration by a multidisciplinary panel:

Generic measures

1. SF-36
2. SF-12
3. EQ-5D

HF-specific measures

4. MLHFQ (Minnesota Living with Heart Failure Questionnaire)
5. KCCQ (Kansas City Cardiomyopathy Questionnaire)

The multidisciplinary panel were favourable toward the SF-36 as a generic measure of health status and the MLHFQ as a heart failure-specific measure. They felt that neither instrument should be used in isolation if the full range of patient experience is to be captured. Having in mind an overall strategy of a generic and condition-specific measure being used in combination to assess complementary aspects of health status, and also having in mind the need for an approach that reduces the volume of questions and likely burden of responding, the current review recommends the combination of EQ-5D and MLHFQ for use in potentially large-scale population studies. The multidisciplinary panel commented on the ease of use of EQ-5D. The simplicity and the brevity of the EQ-5D make it likely that it will not adversely influence response rates.

(Mackintosh *et al.*, 2009)

ACTIVITY 5.3

The results of the national (UK) pilot study on PROMs carried out in the period from April 2009 to August 2010 showed a participation rate of 66.0 per cent for preoperative questionnaires and a return rate of 72.7 per cent for postoperative questionnaires. A total of 95.8 per cent of hip replacement respondents and 91.7 per cent of knee replacement respondents recorded joint-related improvements following their operation. In all, 83.7 per cent of varicose vein respondents recorded varicose vein-related improvements following their operation.

A total of 87.4 per cent of hip replacement respondents and 77.9 per cent of knee replacement respondents recorded an increase in their general health following their operation compared to 52.1 per cent for varicose veins and 49.6 per cent for groin hernias. Some 61.4 per cent of hip replacement respondents and 50.2 per cent of knee replacement respondents recorded an increase in their current state of general health marked on a VAS compared to 40.4 per cent for patients undergoing surgery for varicose veins and 38.2 per cent for those having repair of groin hernias.

Look up the PROMs on the website: **www.ic.nhs.uk/proms**

- What are the main components of a PROM questionnaire?
- What specific outcome measures were used for each condition? What are these measures measuring in particular?
- What is the generic measure of general health which is used? Why do you think patients undergoing hip and knee replacement showed greater increases in their general health than those undergoing varicose vein removal or hernia repair?
- What uses could a clinical commissioning group have for PROMs information?

Comment

A PROM questionnaire has seven components. In addition to patient details and the consent form, there are three important tools for measuring the outcomes. These are the clinical assessment, e.g. Oxford hip score, and the generic health status measures using the EQ-5D profile and the EQ-5D VAS.

The clinical assessment is measured by patients' response to a series of questions about their condition. Three instruments used in the PROMs programme are the Oxford hip and knee scores and the Aberdeen varicose vein questionnaire score. These assess the severity of symptoms (such as pain) and the impact on functionality or quality of life.

The EQ-5D index score is based on a combination of five key criteria concerning general health and the EQ VAS score gives a score between 0 and 100. The reason that the joint replacement patients showed greater impact of the operation on their generic health or quality of life probably relates to the degree of pain associated with joint disease, and the impact, say through immobility, on their daily lives.

PROMs information could be used to assess the appropriateness of referrals to secondary care and to empower commissioners, e.g. establish the quality of services primary care trust commissioners are contracting with the provider.

National outcomes frameworks

The White Paper, *Equity and Excellence: Liberating the NHS,* published in July 2010, set out an ambition to drive the improvement of healthcare outcomes as the primary purpose of the NHS (Department of Health, 2010a, p22). The outcome goals were viewed as providing a means by which patients, the public and Parliament could hold the Secretary of State for Health to account for the overall performance of the NHS. They were also seen as providing a mechanism by which the Secretary of State can hold commissioning bodies to account for securing improved health outcomes for patients through the commissioning process. As well as being a mechanism for accountability it was intended that the NHS Outcomes Framework would act as a catalyst for driving up quality across all NHS services (Department of Health, 2010a).

The principles used in the development of the NHS Outcomes Framework were:

- accountability and transparency;
- balanced;
- focused on what matters to patients and healthcare professionals;
- promoting excellence and equality;
- focused on outcomes that the NHS can influence but working in partnership with other public services where required;
- internationally comparable;
- evolving over time.

The Framework is structured around five high-level outcome domains:

1. Preventing people from dying prematurely
   This domain will capture how successfully the NHS is in reducing the number of avoidable deaths.

2. Enhancing quality of life for people with long-term conditions
   This domain will capture how successfully the NHS is supporting people with long-term conditions to live as normal a life as possible.

3. Helping people to recover from episodes of ill health or following injury
   This domain will capture how people recover from ill health or injury and, wherever possible, how it can be prevented.

4. Ensuring that people have a positive experience of care
   This domain looks at the importance of providing a positive experience of care for patients, service users and carers.

5. Treating and caring for people in a safe environment and protecting them from avoidable harm
   This domain explores patient safety and its importance in terms of quality of care to deliver better health outcomes.

A menu of indicators has been set for each domain, some of which are readily available, and others which will need development. There is a specific set of public health outcomes which includes indicators such as school readiness on the one hand, and others reflecting the social determinants of health as well as the expected mortality rates (Department of Health, 2011b).

Chapter summary

In this chapter we have looked at two main types of outcome – mortality rates and health status measures. The problems of measuring and interpretation are discussed, showing the relative limitations of these types of measure.

However the strengths of using outcome measures as the ultimate way of describing and measuring quality are also clear. You will now know where to look for guidance on outcomes, and how to understand commonly used measures. This will enable you to promote an approach which consistently focuses on the outcomes of the interventions on which we spend our resources so that the most impact can be achieved.

GOING FURTHER

There are a number of websites which are worth browsing:

Association of Public Health Observatories (**www.apho.org.uk**)
> *This is a source of reference material on outcomes measurement and access to outcomes analyses. Look at the various technical briefings.*

National End of Life Care Intelligence Network (**www.endoflifecare-intelligence. org.uk/home.aspx**)
> *The reports will help you understand key aspects of local palliative and terminal care services provision. For example, the report on variations in place of death in England is interesting and raises important issues.*

Quality Observatories (**www.qualityobservatory.nhs.uk**)
> *This provides a source of comparative outcomes data and reports.*

chapter 6

Intelligent Application: Defining the 'So-Whats'

John Harvey

Meeting the Public Health Competences

This chapter will help you to evidence the following competences for public health (Public Health Skills and Career Framework):

- Level 5(2): Analyse routine data on health and wellbeing and needs using basic analytical techniques;
- Level 5(5): Interpret data on health and wellbeing within own area of expertise or practice;
- Level 5(6): Communicate and disseminate findings on the health and wellbeing of a population to others;
- Level 5(a): Knowledge of the links between, and relative importance of, the determinants of health and wellbeing and needs;
- Level 5(d): Understanding of the relevance and use of measures of socioeconomic deprivation in population health and wellbeing analysis;
- Level 6(3): Assess the implications of surveillance and assessment data relating to a defined population and recommend appropriate response(s);
- Level 6(c): Understanding of strengths, uses, interpretation and limitations of various types of data relating to health and wellbeing, needs and outcomes;
- Level 6(d): Understanding of links between, and relative importance of, the various determinants of health and wellbeing and needs;
- Level 6(e): Understanding of the concept and nature of inequalities in health and wellbeing (including use of social deprivation indices);
- Level 7(1): Assess and describe the health and wellbeing and needs of specific populations and the inequities in health and wellbeing experienced by populations, communities and groups;
- Level 8(3): Translate findings about health and wellbeing and needs into appropriate recommendations for action, policy decisions and service commissioning, delivery and provision.

This chapter will also assist you in demonstrating the following National Occupational Standards for public health:

- Analyse data and information about health and wellbeing and/or stressors to health and wellbeing (PHP04);

- Interpret data and information about health and wellbeing and/or stressors to health and wellbeing (PHP05);
- Draft and structure communications about health and wellbeing and/or stressors to health and wellbeing (PHP06);
- Collect and link data and information about the health and wellbeing and related needs of a defined population (PHP10);
- Advise others on data and information related to health and wellbeing and/or stressors to health and wellbeing and its uses (PHP10);
- Manage, analyse, interpret and communicate information, knowledge and statistics about needs and outcomes of health and wellbeing (PHS02).

This chapter will also be useful in demonstrating Standard 6 of the Public Health Practitioner Standards.

Standard 6

Obtain, verify, analyse and interpret data and/or information to improve the health and wellbeing outcomes of a population/community/group – demonstrating:

a. knowledge of the importance of accurate and reliable data/information and the anomalies that might occur;
b. knowledge of the main terms and concepts used in epidemiology and the routinely used methods for analysing quantitative and qualitative data;
c. ability to make valid interpretations of the data and/or information and communicate these clearly to a variety of audiences.

Overview

This chapter aims to provide a practical view of the use of measures of health and wellbeing to influence decision making, whether by commissioners or in a local strategic partnership. The chapter focuses on specific technical methods for using data in decision making, which you should be familiar with and about which you may want to learn more (see further reading suggestions at the end of this chapter). The ultimate focus is the strategic objective of reducing the gap between the measures of health seen in the communities with the worst and best health.

After reading this chapter you will be able to:

- advise others on data and information relating to health and wellbeing and/or stressors to health and wellbeing and its uses;
- communicate data and information about health and wellbeing and related needs of a defined population;
- influence decision making about population health and wellbeing through the presentation, communication and dissemination of data and analysis of health and wellbeing and needs;
- understand the concept and nature of inequalities in health and wellbeing.

Introduction

The key to effective public health practice is not sophisticated data handling but providing practical and evidence-based solutions which can be recognised as both useful and do-able. This book is about measuring health and wellbeing, so this chapter is not about public health interventions, nor a detailed description of health inequalities. Instead the focus is on the practical reality of turning data into intelligence and intelligence into proposals to improve health and wellbeing that make sense to commissioners. This chapter introduces you to different ways of using the measures we have discussed in earlier chapters in a rational contribution to investment in health. Figure 6.1 sets out a schema for achieving the ultimate goal – improving health and wellbeing so that the gaps between the communities with the best and worst health are narrowed. At the heart of the framework is inequalities and scrutiny of inequalities in health and wellbeing in terms of how we can measure the impact of any intervention in terms of narrowing the gap between the communities with the best and worst health. The framework begins with a consideration of the data, interpreting what it means, the implications for the health and wellbeing of the population, the potential interventions and impact of the range of options available measured in terms of outcomes.

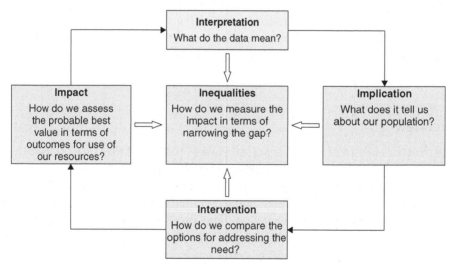

Figure 6.1 5 I's of intelligent need assessment

We will take each box in turn and describe a specific technique or resource to help answer the key question.

Interpretation: What do the data mean?

The first two chapters of this book emphasised some of the limitations of commonly used measures, and the importance of understanding how the data are collected and analysed. Interpreting data is about putting the right strength on the conclusions (if any) to be drawn from any given indicator. There are three fallacies to be aware of.

Activity does not necessarily indicate need, but may be a proxy for need

The number of people attending a service or undergoing a procedure is determined by demand, filtered through a professional referrer in the case of specialised services, and supply. The prevalence of autism spectrum disorder is commonly estimated as being around one child in 100. This is based on children known to services with that label (or better, diagnosis). A recent community survey in Korea puts the figure as two and a half times as much (Kim *et al.*, 2011).

Comparisons and benchmarks

Many indicators are presented in relation to a selected norm, often a regional or national average. Is the value for population A significantly worse or better than the national average? This can be presented in a RAG format (red for significantly worse, amber for neither better nor worse and green for significantly better). Other formats put the value in a centile group, usually in four (25 per cent) or five (20 per cent) groupings. Being in the top centile group or significantly better than average is desirable. This is a performance management approach rather than a need assessment. The obvious fact is that, however much improvement takes place, there will always be those above and below the average, and there will always be a centile distribution. The same problem is created by standardised ratios, where 100 is the 'average' value and above or below is seen as good depending on the indicator.

A different approach is to try to establish a benchmark or 'gold standard' as the target. For example, in one primary care trust in England the directly standardised mortality rates from cardiovascular disease (CVD) for persons under 75 are similar to the national rate, and decreased by 57.5 per cent between 1995–97 and 2007–09. The directly standardised rate per 100,000 for 2007–09 was 69.1 but the England best was 46.3 per 100,000 (**http://www.sepho.org.uk/CVDprofiles.aspx**). The directly standardised rate for another country such as France, which has lower rates of ischaemic heart disease, will be lower. So the issue becomes not how to be better than average in the country but how to reduce the rates radically, aiming at the national or international best rate.

Hotspots

Any mapping of socioeconomic indicators such as the index of multiple deprivation, or the child poverty index, by ward or by super output area will show 'hotspots'.

These are areas of greatest socioeconomic deprivation and almost every indicator of health and wellbeing can be predicted to be worse in those areas than in the least deprived communities.

This is seen in Figure 6.2, where the map on the left shows index of multiple deprivation 2004 by super output area in decicentiles (where darker is more deprived) and the map on the right shows Accident and Emergency attendance rates per 100,000 (where darker is greater). The 'hotspots' are immediately identifiable; however it is important to recognise and be aware that not all vulnerable people are in the obviously deprived areas.

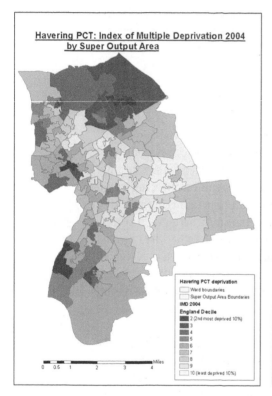 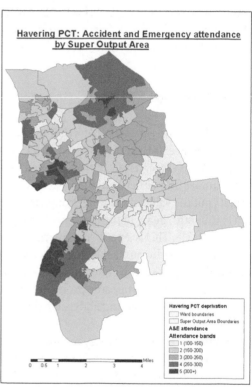

Figure 6.2 Maps of a London borough by super output area (SOA), showing the index of multiple deprivation (IMD) and attendance rates at Accident and Emergency (A&E). PCT, primary care trust

Source: Department of Public Health, NHS Havering.

In many communities, even at small area level, vulnerable neighbourhoods or households may be below the radar of aggregated data. This is especially true of small ethnic groups, which may be found in a few households in a district, and are recent immigrants from areas such as Eastern Europe or sub-Saharan Africa. In this case local intelligence (for example, from data provided at the primary school level) is needed.

Case Study: Using the joint strategic needs assessment (JSNA)

One London borough looked at the rates for hospital admissions for children and young people (aged 18 and under). They found they had a lower rate of admissions for certain conditions: diabetes, gastrointestinal conditions and emergency admissions for lower respiratory tract infections (LRTIs). This was compared to England and London rates. In the case of emergency admissions for LRTI, the borough could be ranked in comparison with other London boroughs 16th out of 31.

On the other hand the same borough had a higher rate of admissions for epilepsy and asthma. The rate for epilepsy was reported as the highest of the London boroughs. Hospitalisations for alcohol-related conditions in persons aged 18 years and under in the borough were lower than the London and England rates but high compared with other boroughs with similar populations.

This scenario raises two key issues: first, how helpful is the admission rate for any specified condition and second, how helpful is the comparison? The need-based rate is the actual prevalence of diabetes (or asthma), which will give an indicative order of actual numbers of children and young people who require some level of service. The admission rate will depend on the availability of expert help outside hospital – a community specialist diabetic nurse, say, or a general practitioner with specialist interest and skills. In considering how helpful the comparison is the same argument is relevant – if the care pathway for any of these conditions is fully resourced then the expectation is that the probability of needing a hospital admission will be reduced. So the key question would be whether an audit of the care pathway would show that all the standards of care are being met.

The author of this JSNA recommended that a detailed analysis of emergency admissions take place to identify those that could have been prevented through improving primary and community initiatives. This is reasonable, if it hasn't already been done. The aim would be to analyse emergency admissions for 0–4-year-olds and 5–19-year-olds to identify preventable admissions to hospital and how the care pathway is being implemented. A wider audit of the care pathways for each condition should be planned too.

Implication: What does it tell us about our population?

The discussion above points to the need to turn data into more than information; rather to turn data into knowledge of the population's needs. The inescapable fact will be the differences between the health and wellbeing of those who are in work, own their house, have attained a high level of educational attainment and earn better than average incomes from those who haven't and don't. This is the health inequalities challenge which has been highlighted (yet again) by the report *Fair Society, Healthy Lives* (Marmot, 2010).

The implication is that interventions should be targeted at the neighbourhoods with the highest levels of deprivation. From an NHS perspective these are usually based on a medical model of need and service and currently with a focus on lifestyle change, for example, and making services such as community midwifery more accessible. An example of this approach is the Sure Start programme.

Sure Start was a government initiative in England which aimed to give children the best possible start in life. This was to be achieved through improvement of child care, early education, health and family support. The programme was originally intended to support families from pregnancy until children were 4 years old and brought together Family Support, including support and advice on parenting, and targeted services with community child health services, such as antenatal and post-natal support, information and guidance on breastfeeding, health and nutrition, smoking cessation support, speech and language therapy and other specialist support. Sure Start programmes were established in disadvantaged areas.

At this stage we usually find that we only know what is wrong or pathological about a given population, and nothing or very little about the strengths of the constituent communities. This is why the Health and Social Care Act (2012) places the 'enhanced' JSNA at the heart of local commissioning. One aspect of an enhanced JSNA is the understanding of local communities and there is an alternative approach which will give rich relevant information. This approach is known as asset mapping and will provide the knowledge needed to help the people living in a neighbourhood to tackle their own issues. Without the complementary knowledge we cannot fully understand the implications of the high-level analysis for the population.

What is an asset?

A health asset has been defined as:

> *any factor or resource which enhances the ability of individuals, communities and populations to maintain and sustain health and wellbeing. These assets can operate at the level of the individual, family or community as protective and promoting factors to buffer against life's stresses.*

(Morgan and Ziglio, 2010)

In an influential report (IDeA, 2010) it was argued that taking an asset-based approach could improve community health and wellbeing. This approach puts a value on the capacity, skills, knowledge, connections and potential in a community, i.e. the glass is half-full. The more familiar 'deficit' approach focuses on the problems, needs and deficiencies in a community such as deprivation, illness and health-damaging behaviours, i.e. the glass is half-empty. The problem-based approach leads to solutions which are based on designing services to fill the gaps or fix the problems. This is disempowering but comfortable for professionals who tend to create dependence. The result is that people can become passive recipients of services rather than

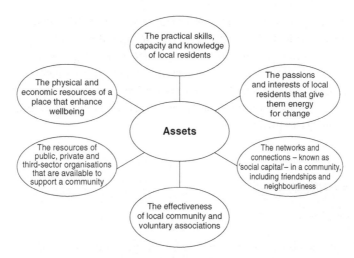

Figure 6.3 Assets identified in *A Glass Half-Full* (IDeA, 2010)

active agents in their own and their families' lives. Figure 6.3 sets out the range of different assets identified in the IDeA report.

The asset approach is a set of values and principles and a way of thinking about the world. While these principles will lead to new kinds of community-based working, they could also be used to refocus many existing council and health service programmes. Characteristics of an asset-based approach are set out in Table 6.1.

Table 6.1 Characteristics of an asset-based approach

Identifies and makes visible the health-enhancing assets in a community

Sees citizens and communities as the co-producers of health and wellbeing, rather than the recipients of services

Promotes community networks, relationships and friendships that can provide caring, mutual help and empowerment

Values what works well in an area

Identifies what has the potential to improve health and wellbeing

Supports individuals' health and wellbeing through self-esteem, coping strategies, resilience skills, relationships, friendships, knowledge and personal resources

Empowers communities to control their futures and create tangible resources such as services, funds and buildings

Asset mapping categorises assets – actual and potential – in six levels:

1. the assets of individuals, such as skills, networks, time;
2. the assets of associations, both formal community organisations or voluntary groups and informal networks like the local boy or girl football team;
3. the assets of organisations, such as parks, or faith buildings;
4. the physical assets of an area, both (green) space and the built environment;
5. the economic assets of an area, such as local shops and new businesses;
6. the cultural assets of an area, such as opportunities for music or art.

Ideally, asset mapping starts with volunteers mapping assets of individuals and of the community. A skilled community organiser supports the community through the process. Asset mapping is most effective when done by a group with an agreed aim. For example, if they want to connect more young girls with non-competitive sport, leisure and fun activities, then associations and other asset holders can respond clearly. In this way a community can amplify and multiply existing resources and promote better involvement.

What's the evidence?

Use of asset mapping

The following is the abstract of an article by Morgan and Ziglio (2007):

Historically, approaches to the promotion of population health have been based on a deficit model. That is, they tend to focus on identifying the problems and needs of populations that require professional resources and high levels of dependence on hospital and welfare services. These deficit models are important and necessary to identify levels of needs and priorities. But they need to be complemented by some other perspectives as they have some drawbacks. Deficit models tend to define communities and individuals in negative terms, disregarding what is positive and works well in particular populations. In contrast 'assets' models tend to accentuate positive capability to identify problems and activate solutions. They focus on promoting salutogenic resources that promote the self esteem and coping abilities of individuals and communities, eventually leading to less dependency on professional services.

Much of the evidence available to policy makers to inform decisions about the most effective approaches to promoting health and to tackling health inequities is based on a deficit model and this may disproportionately lead to policies and practices which disempower the populations and communities who are supposed to benefit from them. An assets approach to health and development embraces a 'salutogenic' notion of health creation and in doing so encourages the full participation of local communities in the health development process.

The asset model presented here aims to revitalise how policy makers, researchers and practitioners think and act to promote a more resourceful approach to tackling health inequities. The model outlines a systematic approach to asset based public health which can provide scientific evidence and best practice on how to maximise the stock of key assets necessary for promoting health. Redressing the balance between the assets and deficit models for evidence based public health could help us to unlock some of the existing barriers to effective action on health inequities. This re-balancing would help in better understanding the factors that influence health and what can be done about them. It would promote a positive and inclusive approach to action.

Read the full article (see references).

Reproduced with permission

ACTIVITY 6.1

Think about the community in which you live, and follow these steps:

1. Get hold of a high-definition map of the area.
2. Define the boundaries of the community.
3. Determine what type of assets to include.
4. Write down the list of partners you would involve in identifying assets.
5. List the assets of groups or organisations, and where they are based or can be accessed.
6. List the physical assets (spaces, facilities, etc.).
7. Organise assets on the map.

Comment

The final picture you will create is a physical map which shows the organisations and physical assets which appear to be accessible to the community. This should include statutory and non-statutory agencies, and community-based organisations. This is fairly straightforward, and may show a geographical pattern where the assets are clustered in or near the community or a much more scattered pattern. What you would want to do next is to determine how far people would see these assets as assets for the community in reality, for example, accessible because they are in reach by walking. The next step then would be to arrange with the partners you listed to talk to residents and to the organisations to determine the patterns of use, and reflect that on the map. There may be some surprises. This will give you a mental map of the area which displays the extent to which the assets you identified are seen truly as assets for the people.

Interventions: How do we compare the options for addressing the need?

In this section we ask the question: 'How do we compare the options for addressing the need?', given we can identify interventions that are judged to be effective in the first place. Broadly speaking, you will find options for intervention in a variety of sources. An intervention may be a single treatment such as a drug, a service such as sexual health service or a programme such as breast screening. All these examples are from a medical model, of course, but there are other options within the social models of health and wellbeing (see Chapter 1), such as parenting programmes in early years, which should be considered.

When trying to identify a long list of possible interventions there are five types of source you may look at. These are:

1. existing (historical) interventions;

2. innovations offered by providers;

3. national policy documents;

4. evidence-based guidance;

5. published case studies.

These sources are compared in Table 6.2.

Table 6.2 Looking for interventions: types of source compared

Source	Description	Strength of evidence base for effectiveness	Likelihood of economic evaluation
Existing (historical) interventions	These are the existing services which are increasingly being subject to evaluation	Often weak, but that does not mean any single intervention is ineffective	Rare
Innovations offered by providers	May present as a case for service development in line with perceived good practice or be genuine innovation	Variable Service developments may have modest to good evidence. Innovations by definition need evaluating	Poor
National policy documents	Are usually contention-led rather than evidence-based with case studies of good practice, typically unevaluated	Poor	Poor
Evidence-based guidance	These include NICE* guidance and other reports from agencies with robust scientific reviews	Good Use of meta-analyses and substantive literature reviews	Good
Published case studies	These may be a research study, case series, or service evaluation published in peer-reviewed journals, or reports of good practice published by agencies such as medical colleges	Variable These studies need to be reviewed critically, but may point to other relevant good evidence	Variable May be good enough to use in prioritisation

* NICE, National Institute for Health and Clinical Excellence

At this stage you will have the long list referred to above. It is (very) unlikely that the local commissioners will have the resources to commission all of that list so a process has to be followed to reduce the list to an affordable group of the most effective interventions (the short list). There are different ways of doing this, but it will involve a method of multi-criteria decision analysis (MCDA). The process is known as prioritisation.

Case Study: Prioritising investments in preventive health

Matrix Insight produced a report for Health England in 2009. Health England is the national reference group for health and wellbeing. The objective of the report is to develop and apply a method for prioritising preventive health interventions. In particular they wanted to develop a method that would be useful and accessible for decision-makers (Matrix Insight, 2009).

The method used to prioritise interventions was MCDA. The approach sought to evaluate interventions according to the number of people who benefit and the distribution of these benefits between population groups, as well as according to their cost-effectiveness, and to rank interventions in order of priority.

The authors used the following steps, which are common to all MCDAs:

- Identifying interventions to evaluate. The interventions included in the analysis had to be of interest to decision-makers and have been the subject of a review of effectiveness and/or cost-effectiveness.
- Identifying criteria against which to evaluate the interventions. The criteria included in the analysis had to be identified by decision-makers and be measurable.

  Five criteria were included in the analysis:

  1. cost-effectiveness: cost per quality-adjusted life year gained, including healthcare costs avoided;
  2. the proportion of the population eligible for the intervention;
  3. the distribution of benefits: the ratio of the proportion of the most disadvantaged 20 per cent of the population eligible for the intervention to the proportion of the population as a whole eligible for the intervention;
  4. affordability: the budget required to fund the intervention if all eligible people received the intervention;
  5. certainty: confidence in the evaluation of the intervention, based on an assessment of the quality of the method and data used in the evaluation.

- Measuring the interventions against the criteria.
- Combining the scores for all criteria to produce an overall assessment of each intervention. Criteria weights were calculated by undertaking a discrete choice experiment to elicit decision-makers' preferences for the criteria.

The final analysis was run for 17 interventions covering the following problem areas: alcohol use, mental health, obesity, smoking cessation and sexually transmitted infections. The use of statins was also included as a benchmark intervention.

Their conclusions included:

- increasing tax on cigarettes and alcohol is the intervention that best meets decision-makers' objectives;
- mass media campaigns and brief interventions delivered by GPs also performed well;
- all interventions outperform the use of statins, other than the interventions included in the analysis aimed at improving mental health.

The case study is about prioritisation. Prioritisation is the process of ranking competing items, such as tasks or potential purchases, in order of importance. Priority setting is a key component of the process of evaluating health interventions in order to decide what investments should be made with limited resources.

A number of explicit criteria and systematic models have been developed since the late 1980s. These models increasingly seek to inform and involve the public.

The process of prioritisation involves the use of agreed criteria to judge relative importance. These criteria are used to score each option. The criteria commonly used do not vary much from organisation to organisation, or country to country. However they also reflect the values of an organisation and may overlap with aspects of an agreed ethical framework.

Underlying the process of prioritisation are three health economics concepts:

1. Resources are limited and must be allocated prudently.

2. Cost–benefit analysis, estimating whether costs are reasonable in relation to expected benefit, will provide information to help discriminate between options.

3. Opportunity costs have to be considered – if £100,000 is spent on option A, then it cannot be spent elsewhere.

The key point of this section is that, in order to put in place effective intervention to address the issues we have agreed with the people in the target population, within available resources, we should use a systematic and transparent process of prioritisation.

Impact: How do we assess the probable best value in terms of outcomes for use of our resources?

In this section we ask questions about the impact of an intervention on the target population. One question is: How do we measure the impact on their health and wellbeing? Another would be: How do we assess the impact in terms of getting the probable best outcomes given the resources available?

There has been considerable interest in the NHS in the concept of high-impact interventions since 2004. The first set of ten high-impact changes was produced after auditing thousands of improvement projects with NHS clinical teams over a number of years. It included making day surgery the normal mode for planned surgery. Similarly, high-impact interventions have been developed in public health. For example, NHS Yorkshire and the Humber produced a guide to integrating high-impact actions into healthcare practice to reduce smoking preconception, during pregnancy and postpartum. One action is about reaching pregnant smokers as soon as possible and throughout pregnancy because of the potential impact on reducing infant mortality. The actions were seen as one means of tackling health inequalities (NHS Yorkshire and the Humber, 2007).

Measuring the impact of interventions on health and wellbeing of specified populations has been discussed in the chapter on outcomes (see Chapter 5). In this context the issue is how to measure consistently before and after an intervention has been implemented. Time series data and cross-sectional data should complement each other. Time series data show the extent and direction of changes over time. On the other hand, cross-sectional data, or those describing various groups within the population, show possible disparities among the groups, and how those are changing over time. The data in the impact assessment should have meaningful disaggregations, such as those by sex, age and ethnicity, among others. The answer to what impact we are making will be through judicious use of the kinds of outcome measures we have described. This links to the health inequality tool (for measuring the gap), which is highlighted in the next section.

The second question is: How do we assess the impact in terms of getting the probable best outcomes given the resources available? This can be tackled using marginal analysis – a health economic technique. Not everyone agrees that health needs assessment (HNA) is the most effective way of identifying health priorities. Some health economists have argued that there are disadvantages in assessing total needs when setting priorities. A fundamental premise of health economists is that all needs cannot be met due to the scarcity of resources. The main problem in using information on total needs for setting priorities is the implication that priorities will be determined by the amount of need or the size of the problem. In their view HNA does not take sufficient account of the limited resources available. They argue that the focus for setting priorities is at the 'margin' – making changes to the way in which scarce resources are allocated to maximise health gain.

Marginal analysis is the economists' alternative approach to HNA. The starting point is the current distribution of resources between different services or different parts of the care pathway for specific conditions. Marginal analysis then looks at the effect of incremental changes to the way in which resources could be allocated in order to gain the most health benefit (the impact).

Marginal analysis is based on three basic economic principles.

1. Resources are scarce relative to need, which means that choices have to be made.

2. Decisions on where to allocate resources (priorities) should be made on the basis of explicit criteria. One criterion is efficiency, which is about maximising the benefit from available resources.

3. Allocating resources to one service means that this resource is not available for other services. The benefit that the resources might have produced in another service is the opportunity cost.

These economic principles underpin the health economic framework for priority setting – programme budgeting and marginal analysis (PBMA). This framework can be described by asking five questions about the use of resources.

1. What resources are available?
2. In what ways are these resources currently allocated?
3. What are the main candidates for more resources and what would be their level of effectiveness?
4. Are there any areas of care which could be provided to the same level of effectiveness but with fewer resources, so releasing those resources to fund candidates from point 3? (technical efficiency).
5. Are there any areas of care which, despite being effective, should receive fewer resources because a proposal from point 3 is more cost-effective? (allocative efficiency).

If you are interested in learning more you can access a guide on the Map of Medicine website (**www.mapofmedicine.com**) by looking at the healthcare management section. There is a step-by-step guide to carrying out a PBMA exercise.

What's the evidence?

Use of PBMA

Mitton and Donaldson undertook a study in 1999 to assess the use of PBMA over the previous 25 years in the health sector. At that time, no formal evaluation of this framework had been conducted. The aims of this study were to categorise previous PBMA exercises systematically and determine the impact of PBMA in regional health authorities (RHAs) internationally.

The study was undertaken by contacting 30 authors of grey literature and published papers on PBMA, and an additional six economists with research interests in PBMA. They were surveyed with a mailed questionnaire. Previous exercises were categorised and details of the short- and long-term impacts of the framework were obtained.

The results showed that the PBMA framework was identified as having been used 78 times in 59 RHAs. For the exercises where longer-term impact was known, the approach was viewed as having had a positive impact, as defined by the setting of priorities or shifting of resources, in 59 per cent of cases and continued to be used in at least 52 per cent of the RHAs. The primary reasons why PBMA was discontinued included personnel changes and lack of internal 'champions'.

The authors concluded that:

> contrary to popular perception, there has been widespread diffusion of PBMA in RHAs internationally and, overall, the impact of this approach has been positive. Although there is general agreement on the validity of the economic principles underlying PBMA, addressing managerial issues would seem to be central to successful implementation in a given region.
>
> (Mitton and Donaldson, 2001)

The success of a systematic approach to the use of the total resource is in part dependent on an understanding of the specific impact within the target population terms of any given intervention. The case study below illustrates the kind of analysis which is needed to take this process forward.

Case Study: Risk factors and public health interventions in Denmark

A study in Denmark published in 2008 looked at the health and economic aspects of risk factors and the impact of interventions. Figure 6.4 illustrates the assessment of impact you would use to undertake marginal analysis. It shows the predicted reduction in mortality from ischaemic heart disease 15 years after initiation of two different interventions to reduce physical inactivity and illustration of the significance of the choice of relative risk (Juel et al., 2008).

Intervention implemented gradually over a 10-year period	Reduction in mortality from ischaemic heart disease among Danes aged less than 65 years (%)	
	Men	Women
Scenario 1		
'No sedentary persons A' All sedentary persons (RR = 1.9) become slightly physically active (RR = 1.7)	3	5
'No sedentary persons B' * All sedentary persons (RR = 3.0) become slightly physically active (RR = 2.0)	7	10
Scenario 2 All persons who do not perform hard training exercise and competitive sports raise their level of physical activity by one step relative to the categories:	20	20
– Perform hard training exercise and competitive sports (RR = 1)		
– Moderately physically active (RR = 1.4)		
– Slightly physically active (RR = 1.7)		
– Sedentary (RR = 1.9)		

Figure 6.4 The impact of interventions

* In scenario 1B the relative risks (RR) are increased arbitrarily to show the impact of RR on the model.

Health inequalities

Throughout this book we have kept coming back to the differences in health and wellbeing which we can measure between different population groups and geographical populations. This is the problem known as health inequalities and is a reflection of the strata of factors such as educational achievement and income levels in society. As stated in the first chapter, the Marmot (2010) report *Fair Society, Healthy Lives* sets out some priorities for tackling the root causes.

In this chapter we have focused on intelligent application of the knowledge we have through the myriad of measures available to us. We need to interpret the data carefully to draw the true implications. Having identified neighbourhoods or communities which are vulnerable we want to understand their needs at a deeper level. Asset mapping gives an approach which engages people and focuses on the aspects which contribute to the resilience of a community and should be built on to improve health and wellbeing. In addressing inequalities we need to apply our understanding of the cost-effectiveness of possible interventions to choose the best options within the resource available. This needs a prioritisation process, and then we have to use the best knowledge available to predict and measure the impact so that our investment gains the most benefit. In health inequality terms this is often seen as narrowing the gap. There is a tool for measuring inequalities produced by the Association of Public Health Observatories (APHO). In addition the APHO now has a profile for local authorities of ten so-called Marmot indicators. An example is the indicator of inequality in disability-free life expectancy (DFLE).

DFLE is the average number of years a person could expect to live without an illness or health problem that limits his or her daily activities. This indicator is the slope index of inequality in DFLE. It summarises the social inequality in DFLE within each local authority. The slope index of inequality represents the gap in years of DFLE between the least and most deprived areas within the local authority, based on a statistical analysis of the relationship between DFLE and deprivation scores across the whole authority. In this index the higher the value, the greater the inequality within the local authority.

The Department of Health commissioned the APHO to produce a toolkit to contribute to the achievement of the national health inequalities Public Service Agreement target: *Reduce health inequalities by 10% by 2010 as measured by infant mortality and life expectancy at birth.*

The London Health Observatory developed the toolkit. Its purpose is to:

- quantify the current life expectancy gap at birth within local authority areas, and between spearhead local authorities and England;

- quantify the diseases contributing to the life expectancy gap;

- model the effect of four high-impact interventions on closing the life expectancy gap.

The online tool will give a breakdown of the life expectancy gap for your area (local authority) and compare the worst and best small areas within the population. Figure 6.5 shows one facet of the outputs from the tool.

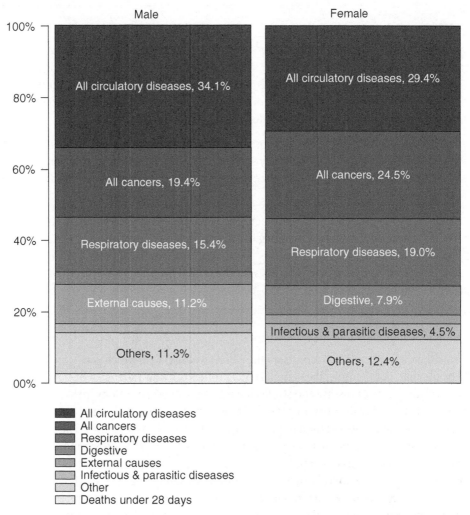

Figure 6.5 Breakdown of life expectancy gap between the most deprived quintile (MDQ) and the England average by cause of death for one local authority

---

ACTIVITY 6.2

The London Health Observatory tool for reducing inequalities identified key factors in relation to the gap between infant mortality rates for mothers from routine/manual households and all births. Some of the factors are smoking (12 per cent of the gap), obesity (9 per cent) and sudden unexplained deaths in infants (8 per cent). Poverty makes a measurable but small contribution. Given these factors, what interventions would you include on a long list to reduce the infant mortality rates? How would you decide what would go on your short list? See if you can find the evidence to make an assessment against whatever criteria you have chosen for one or two interventions.

> **Comment**
>
> First, you should identify what factors are associated with poor infant health and high infant mortality. These include a range of factors, such as women living in families where both partners are unemployed, women living in the most deprived areas, late booking and poor attenders at antenatal clinics, maternal age, women who are drug and/or alcohol users. Your long list will reflect these factors.
>
> Second, set some criteria for assessing which interventions will have the most impact. This will include the cost-effectiveness, magnitude of health benefit and impact on infant health, and the impact on inequality. The data above help with the assessment of that criterion.
>
> Finally, having researched the evidence (the National Institute for Health and Clinical Excellence website (**www.nice.org.uk**) may help you), you can select four or five options for investment based on the criteria you selected. This short list will probably include enhanced services to help mothers quit smoking, and effective strategies for weight reduction preconception.

There are other helpful tools and reports on the APHO website, with which you should be familiar. For example, the national CVD profiles provide a snapshot of key issues relating to heart disease and stroke, including incidence, mortality, risk factors, treatments and costs. They are intended to inform commissioning and planning decisions to tackle CVD and improve the health of local communities. The profiles have a summary spine chart showing a number of selected indicators; a more detailed profile; and an interactive atlas.

Another example is Technical Briefing 8, on prevalence modelling. This briefing discusses the need for prevalence modelling and provides an overview of various methods of generating estimates of the prevalence of diseases or risk factors in local populations.

> **Chapter summary**
>
> This chapter has looked at four aspects – interpretation, implications, interventions and impact – of applying measures intelligently in order to understand the health and wellbeing of a population, to explore the needs at neighbourhood level and decide on cost-effective interventions. The chapter also discusses ways of measuring the impact, especially on narrowing the gap in inequalities. There is a wealth of good information and tools to use the data in a way that is relevant and credible. We point you to some of those resources. The next step is to start using them!

GOING FURTHER

Austin, D (2007) *Priority Setting: An Overview*. London: The Primary Care Trust Network, The NHS Confederation.
This report is part of a series on managing scarcity in healthcare, published by the NHS Confederation. It sets out the principles of prioritisation and gives guidance on how to establish a framework for prioritisation.

IDeA (2010) *A Glass Half-Full: How an Asset Approach Can Improve Community Health and Well-Being.* London: IDeA.
This is an excellent introduction to the subject, making the case for asset mapping as a vital approach to community development and providing practical techniques for undertaking the work.

Matrix Insight (2009). *Prioritising Investments in Preventative Health.* Report produced for Health England. London: Matrix Insight. Accessed at: **http://www.healthengland.org/health_england_publications.htm**
This represents one approach to producing evidence in order to inform decision making. It is useful to look at the methodology and to think through the validity and implications of the ranking of the intervention. In addition the report refers to an online tool to allow interaction with the analysis.

APHO has a number of very useful short reports. Part 5 of JSNA – the APHO Resource Pack is called Measuring Health Inequalities (APHO, 2008). It gives good illustrations of the technical issues in describing the differences between population groups. Available online at: **www.yhpho.org.uk/resource/item.aspx?RID=9957**. *Yorkshire and Humber Public Health Observatory lead on health economics for the APHO. On their website there is a report entitled Road Testing Programme Budgeting and Marginal Analysis (PBMA) in Three English Regions: Hull (Diabetes), Newcastle (CAHMS), Norfolk (Mental Health). This explains how the project to undertake PBMA was carried out and describes the outputs. Available online at:* **www.yhpho. org.uk/default.aspx?RID=8478**

References

Anderson RT, Aaronson, NK and Wilkin, D (1993) Critical review of the international assessments of health-related quality of life. *Quality of Life Research*, 2:369–395.

APHO (The Association of Public Health Observatories) (2008) *JSNA – The APHO Resource Pack, Part 5: Measuring Health Inequalities*. Accessed at: http://www.apho.org.uk/resource

APHO (The Association of Public Health Observatories) (2010a) Health profiles. Accessed at www.apho.org.uk

APHO (The Association of Public Health Observatories) (2010b) *Dying to Know: How to Interpret and Investigate Hospital Mortality Measures.* Accessed at www.apho.org.uk

Badia, X, Schiaffino, A, Alonso, J and Herdman, M (1998) Using the EuroQol 5-D in the Catalan general population: feasibility and construct validity. *Quality of Life Research* 7:311–322.

Barlow, C and Castilla-Sanchez, F (2012) Occupational noise exposure and regulatory adherence in music venues in the United Kingdom. *Noise and Health*, 14:86–90.

Bowling, A (2000) *Research Methods in Health*. Buckingham: Open University Press.

Bradshaw, J (1972) A taxonomy of social need. *New Society*, March:640–643.

Brambleby, P and Fordham, R (2003) What is PBMA? Available at: www.medicine.ox.ac.uk/bandolier/painres/download/whatis/pbma.pdf (accessed August 2012).

Bridgewater, B (2005) Mortality data in adult cardiac surgery for named surgeons: retrospective examination of prospectively collected data on coronary artery surgery and aortic valve replacement. *BMJ*, 330: 506–510.

British Lung Foundation (2007) *Invisible Lives. Chronic Obstructive Pulmonary Disease (COPD) – Finding the Missing Millions*. London: British Lung Foundation.

Brooks, R, Jendteg, S, Lindgren, B, Persson, U and Björk, S (1991) EuroQol: health-related quality of life measurement. Results of the Swedish questionnaire exercise. *Health Policy*, 18:37–48.

Cavanagh, S and Chadwick, K (2005) *Health Needs Assessment.* London: Health Development Agency.

CDC (2010) *Overview of Public Health Surveillance.* Epidemiology Program Office, Centers for Disease Control and Prevention. Accessed at: www.cdc.gov/osels/ph_surveillance/nndss/phs/files/overview.ppt

Codman, EA (1934) *The Shoulder. Rupture of the Supraspinatus Tendon and Other Lesions In or About the Subacromial Bursa.* Privately published 1934. Reprinted: Malabar, FL: Kreige, 1965.

Dahlgren, G and Whitehead, M (1991) *Policies and Strategies to Promote Social Equity in Health.* Stockholm: Stockholm Institute for Future Studies.

Department for Children, Schools and Families and Department of Health (2009) *Securing Better Health for Children and Young People Through World Class Commissioning. A Guide to Support Delivery of Healthy Lives, Brighter Futures: The Strategy for Children and Young People's Health.* London: DFCS and DoH.

Department of Health (2007a) *The Commissioning Framework for Health and Wellbeing.* London: DoH.

Department of Health (2007b) *Guidance on Joint Strategic Needs Assessment.* London: DoH.

Department of Health (2008) UK Public Health Skills and Career Framework: Multidisciplinary/Multi-agency/Multi-professional. London: Department of Health, Public Health Resource Unit, Skills for Health. www.sph.nhs.uk/sphfiles/PHSkills-CareerFramework_Launchdoc_April08.pdf (accessed April 2011)

Department of Health (2010a) *Equity and Excellence: Liberating the NHS – An Outcomes Framework.* London: Department of Health. Available online at: www.dh.gov.uk/en/Consultations/Liveconsultations/DH_117583

Department of Health (2010b) *The Mid Staffordshire NHS Foundation Trust Inquiry.* London: Department of Health.

Department of Health (2010c) *Transparency in Outcomes – A Framework for the NHS.* A consultation paper. London: DoH.

Department of Health (2011a) *Joint Strategic Needs Assessments and Joint Health and Wellbeing Strategies Explained – Commissioning for Populations.* London: DoH.

Department of Health (2011b) *The National Outcomes Framework 2012/13.* London: Department of Health.

Department of Health (2012) *Draft Guidance on Joint Strategic Needs Assessments and Joint Health and Wellbeing Strategies.* London: DoH.

Donabedian, A (1966) Evaluating the quality of medical care. *Milbank Memorial Fund Quarterly,* 44:166–206.

Donabedian, A (1989) The end results of health care: Ernest Codman's contribution to quality assessment and beyond. *Milbank Q,* 67:233–256.

Elkheir R (2007) *Health Needs Assessment: A Practical Approach.* Available online at: www.sjph.net.sd/files/vol2i2p81-88.pdf

Ereaut, G and Whiting, R (2008) *What Do We Mean by 'Wellbeing'? And Why Might It Matter?* Research report no. DCSF-RW073. London: Linguistic Landscapes.

Flowers, J (2007) *Statistical Process Control Methods in Public Health Intelligence.* Technical briefing no. 2. York: Association of Public Health Observatories.

Francis, R (2010) *The Mid Staffordshire NHS Foundation Trust Inquiry. Independent Inquiry into Care Provided by Mid Staffordshire NHS Foundation Trust January 2005–March 2009,* vol I. London: The Stationery Office. Available online at: www.midstaffsinquiry.com/assets/docs/Inquiry_Report-Vol1.pdf

Frommer, M, Rubin G and Lyle, D (1992) The NSW Health Outcomes program. *NSW Public Hlth Bull* 3: 135–137.

Goldberg, DP (1972) *The Detection of Psychiatric Illness by Questionnaire.* London: Oxford University Press.

Gordon, D, Lloyd, L and Heslop, P (2001) *Jersey Health Survey.* Townsend Centre for International Poverty Research. Bristol: University of Bristol.

Gough, I (1992) What are human needs? in Percy-Smith, J and Sanderson, I (eds) *Understanding Local Needs.* London: Institute for Public Policy Research.

Graham, H and Power, C (2004) *Childhood Disadvantage and Adult Health: A Lifecourse Framework.* London: Health Development Agency.

Gray, L, Merlo, J, Mindell, J, Hallqvist, J, Tafforeau, J, O'Reilly, D, Regidor, E *et al.* (2012) International differences in self-reported health measures in 33 major metropolitan areas in Europe. *Eur J Public Health,* 22:40–47.

Gustafsson, PE, Persson, M and Hammarstrom, A (2011) Life course origins of the metabolic syndrome in middle-aged women and men: the role of socio-economic status and metabolic risk factors in adolescence and early adulthood. *Ann Epidemiol,* 21:103–110.

Hall, DMB (ed) (1989) *Health for All Children.* Report of the Joint Working Party on Child Health Surveillance. Oxford: Oxford University Press.

Hooper, J and Longworth, P (2002) *Health Needs Assessment Workbook.* London: Health Development Agency.

Huber, M, Knottnerus, JA, Green, L, van der Horst, H, Jadad, AR, Kromhout, D, Leonard, B *et al.* (2011) How should we define health? *BMJ,* 343:7817. Available online at: www.bmj.com.libezproxy.open.ac.uk/content/343/bmj. d4163 (accessed 20 August 2012).

IDeA (2010) *A Glass Half-Full: How an Asset Approach Can Improve Community Health and Well-Being.* London: IDeA.

Johnson, JA and Coons, SJ (1998) Comparison of the EQ-5D and SF-12 in an adult US sample. *Quality of Life Research,* 7: 155–166.

Juel, K, Sørensen, J and Brønnum-Hansen, H (2008) Risk factors and public health in Denmark. *Scand J Public Health*, 6:1.

Kim, YS, Leventhal, BL, Koh, YJ, Fombonne, E, Laska, E, Lim, EC, Cheon, KA *et al.* (2011) Prevalence of autism spectrum disorders in a total population sample. *Am J Psychiatry*, 168:904–912.

Kind, P, Dolan, P, Gudex, C and Williams, A (1998) Variations in population health status: results from a United Kingdom national questionnaire survey. *BMJ*, 316:736–741.

Kind, P, Hardman, G and Macran, S (1999) *UK Population Norms for EQ-5D*. The University of York Centre for Health Economics Discussion Paper. York: Centre for Health Economics, p172.

Loane, M, Dolk, H, Bradbury, I and EUROCAT Working Group (2007) Increasing prevalence of gastroschisis in Europe 1980–2002: a phenomenon restricted to younger mothers? *Paediatr Perinatal Epidemiol*, 21:363–369.

Mackintosh, A, Gibbons, E and Fitzpatrick, R (2009) *A Structured Review of Patient-Reported Outcome Measures for People with Heart Failure: An Update*. Patient-reported outcome measurement group. Oxford: University of Oxford.

Marmot, M (2005) Social determinants of health inequalities. *Lancet* 365:1099–1104.

Marmot, M (2010) *Fair Society, Healthy Lives*. The Marmot Review. Accessed at: www.ucl.ac.uk/marmotreview

Matrix Insight (2009) *Prioritising Investments in Preventative Health*. Report produced for Health England. London: Matrix Insight.

Mitton, C and Donaldson, C (2001) Twenty-five years of programme budgeting and marginal analysis in the health sector, 1974–1999. *J Health Serv Res Policy*, 6:239–248.

Morgan, A and Ziglio, E (2007) Revitalising the evidence base for public health: an assets model. *Promotion Education*, 14:17.

Morgan, A and Ziglio, E (2010) Revitalising the public health evidence – an asset model, in Morgan, A, Davies, M and Ziglio, E (eds) *Health Assets in a Global Context: Theory, Methods, Action*. New York: Springer.

Murray, SA (1999) Experiences with 'rapid appraisal' in primary care: involving the public in assessing health needs, orientating staff, and educating medical students. *BMJ*, 318:440. Available online at: www.bmj.com/content/318/7181/440.full (accessed 20 August 2012).

Nacul, LC, Soljak, M and Meade, T (2007) Model for estimating the population prevalence of chronic obstructive pulmonary disease: cross sectional data from the Health Survey for England. *Population Health Metrics*, 5:1–8 (see also: www.pophealthmetrics.com/content/pdf/1478-7954-5-8.pdf; accessed 11 November 2012).

National End of Life Care Intelligence Network (NEoLCIN) (2010) *Variations in Place of Death in England*. NHS End of Life Care Programme. Available online at: www.endoflifecare-intelligence.org.uk/home.aspx

National Information Center on Health Services Research and Health Care Technology (NICHSR) *Health Economics Information Resources: A Self-Study Course*. Available at: www.nlm.nih.gov/nichsr/edu/healthecon/glossary.html

NHS National Services Scotland: Information Services Division (2010) *Data Quality Assurance Assessment of Maternity Data (SMR02) 2008–2009*. Edinburgh: NHS National Services Scotland.

NHS Yorkshire and the Humber (2007) *Reducing Smoking Pre-conception, During Pregnancy and Postpartum: Integrating High Impact Actions into Routine Healthcare Practice*. Leeds: NHS Yorkshire and the Humber, Department of Health.

Nightingale, F (1863) *Notes on Hospitals*. London: Longman, Green, Longman, Roberts and Green.

Overseas Development Institute (2009) Planning tools: problem tree analysis, toolkits. Available online at: www.odi.org.uk/resources/details.asp?id=5258&title =problem-tree-analysis (accessed 12 July 2012).

People and Participation.net. Available at: www.peopleandparticipation.net/ display/Involve/Home (accessed August 2012).

Popay, J, Attree, P, Hornby, D, Milton, B, Whitehead, M, French, B, Kowarzik, U *et al.* (2007) *Community Engagement in Initiatives Addressing the Wider Social Determinants of Health. A Rapid Review of Evidence on Impact, Experience and Process*. Available at http://guidance.nice.org.uk/page.aspx?o=432684

Scadding, JG (1988) Health and disease: what can medicine do for philosophy? *J Med Ethics* 14:118–124.

Social Exclusion Task Force (2007) *Families at Risk: Background on Families with Multiple Disadvantages*. London: Cabinet Office, Social Exclusion Task Force.

Stevens, A and Raftery, J (1994) *Introduction; Health Care Needs Assessment: The Epidemiologically Based Needs Assessment Reviews,* vol 1. Oxford: Radcliffe Medical Press.

Sykes, S (2009) Health needs assessment and the community nurse, in Sines, D, Saunders, M and Forbes-Burford, J (eds) *Community Health Care Nursing*. Chichester: Wiley Blackwell.

The Control of Noise at Work Regulations (2005) Accessed at http://www.legislation. gov.uk/uksi/2005/1643/

Walker, S, Palmer, S and Sculpher, M (2007) The role of NICE technology appraisal in NHS rationing. *Br Med Bull*, 81–82:51–64.

Wickrama, KA, Conger, RD, Wallace, LE and Elder, GH Jr (2003) Linking early social risks to impaired physical health during the transition to adulthood. *J Health Soc Behav*, 44:61–74.

Wilkinson, R and Marmot, M (2003) *The Solid Facts*. Copenhagen: World Health Organization.

World Health Organization (WHO) (1948) Preamble to the Constitution of the World Health Organization as adopted by the International Health Conference, New York, 19 June–22 June 1946; signed on 22 July 1946 by the representatives of 61 States (Official Records of the World Health Organization, no. 2, p. 100) and entered into force on 7 April 1948. New York: WHO. Accessed at: www. who.int/about/definition/en/print.html

World Health Organization (WHO) (1986) The Ottawa Charter for Health Promotion. First International Conference on Health Promotion, Ottawa, November 1986. Accessed at: http://www.who.int/hpr/NPH/docs/ottawa_ charter_hp.pdf

World Health Organization (WHO) (2008a) *Commission on Social Determinants of Health*. Geneva: World Health Organization.

World Health Organization (2008b) *International Health Regulations* (2005), 2nd edition. Geneva: WHO.

World Health Organization (WHO) (2010) *Public Health Surveillance*. Available at: www.who.int/immunization_monitoring/burden/routine_surveillance/en/ index.html (accessed August 2012).

World Health Organization (WHO) (2011) *The WHO STEPwise Approach to Chronic Disease Risk Factor Surveillance (STEPS)*. Geneva: World Health Organization. Available at: www.who.int/chp/steps/en (accessed August 2012).

Wright, J (2001) Assessing health needs, in Pencheon, D, Guest, C, Melzer, D and Gray, JAM (eds) *The Oxford Handbook of Public Health Practice*. Oxford: Oxford University Press.

Wright, J, Williams, R and Wilkinson, JR (1998) Development and importance of health needs assessment. *BMJ*, 316:1310–1313.

Index